The Weight of Words

~~Dieting and Dying~~ Living and Dining

in the

Midwest and Middle East

The Weight of Words

~~Dieting and Dying~~ Living and Dining

in the

Midwest and Middle East

Sandra Humble Johnson

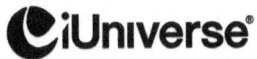

The Weight of Words
~~Dieting and Dying~~ Living and Dining in the Midwest and Middle East

iUniverse books may be ordered through booksellers or by contacting:

iUniverse
1663 Liberty Drive
Bloomington, IN 47403
www.iuniverse.com
844-349-9409

ISBN: 978-1-4401-4523-0 (sc)
ISBN: 978-1-4401-4525-4 (hc)
ISBN: 978-1-4401-4524-7 (e)

Print information available on the last page.

iUniverse rev. date: 06/15/2023

For Brooke,
who is on the adventure with me

I have changed the names of several of the participants in this story, in order to protect their anonymity.

Contents

Prologue: Map

A word weighs more than the flesh of your body. More than your flesh and bones together. And this weight can be joy and elegance or the burden of despair. For a word signifies a pattern in your brain, and it is this pattern, repeated daily, hourly, in your thoughts, that might have caused you to pick up this book. You do not like what you've become in the flesh. You can't walk like you used to. You breathe heavily and try another exercise program. You can't zip up your pants. Your thighs spread thick, pushing the fabric out in lumps at the sides of your dress—like doughnuts that won't go away. You turn sideways in the mirror, sucking it in, pulling up your shoulders, but the lifting of your frame doesn't remedy the stretched, gapping shirt or the straining buttons. Disgusted and fearful, you turn away and think *this can't be happening* or *this time, I'm really going to do it.*

Or perhaps your nagging desire is an adventure not taken.

Just as a word brings that extra flesh, a word can take it away, and just as a word keeps you sitting in your chair, your hand on the remote, with TV tuned in to the travel channel, a word can put you on a plane, studying a map of Paris or Rome. Or maybe even Arabia. A word can create you. I know this because I've used words to shape not only my body but, in tandem, my life—that is, my occupation and my landscape. I've learned that my life rests first in my body. If I don't have this frame in place, strong, able to walk through the day, to climb stairs, to bend over to tie my shoes, or to pull up my panty hose, then I will perpetually seek out systems to clean up, pare down, and set it all right. If I don't have strength, I'll not be able to attend to that next dream, that adventure, that idea that many people dub as the "thing they always wanted to do but didn't get around to," and I will sit in the doctor's office flipping through *Budget Travel*. Words make things happen.

I know this because, nineteen years ago, I changed my mind; that is, I changed the map in my mind. I altered my interior landscape with language. And this vocabulary, selected and habitually used, changed my body, or what I call my immediate exterior landscape. I lost the weight that had haunted me since I was a child. Big thighs in my black band uniform, spreading zipper teeth that caught my skin on the way up, 2× panty hose, and longing, the longing to not live for food—these were all a part of my Ohio life. I was happy in Ohio with my husband, my child, and my job. But the frustration and nagging desire to be slender was always with me—to wear clothes that fell sleekly over my hips, to not react to life by gorging myself with candy bars or casseroles or buttered toast. And then I changed my words.

And then ten years ago, I changed another landscape. I came to the Arabian Peninsula to teach. From West Liberty, Ohio, and its one-block downtown street, to Dubai, and its glittering rows of mirrored towers, I switched my position on the map of the world. And all of this was the result of words. As a professor in a university for Emirati women, I work with language. In a city glittering with Jaguars, Bentleys, and Rolex, I've been given the opportunity to observe a culture far from Ohio, to live with these desert people and observe that all the world moves on the scudding of words across the page and across the mind. This book is a brief record of my reaction to these interior and exterior landscapes, the shifting of language, and the ultimate power of words.

Nancy Drew and the Desert

Jesus with a cell phone, white robe, just ahead, there by the Daniel Hector and Rodeo Drive windows, talking to the air, microphone emerging from the side of his scarf or hood—or what should I call it? He peers in at the sleek cut of a Ralph Lauren jacket and leans down to check out the dull, expensive shine of Italian calf shoes. Up ahead, a batch of Bible Marys cluster around a Starbucks table, lifting caramel lattes to maroon-outlined lips, whispering, and adjusting Gucci sunglasses at the edge of their scarves—or should I say, their wimples? A fleck of rhinestone glitters against the swag of black robe draping from one girl's arm. Her hand, scrolled in mahogany flowers, holds a Nokia cell phone against her cheek. Encrusted with stones, this, too, flashes under the avenue of mall neon. She laughs, clicks her stiletto heels under the table, and looks surreptitiously at the apostles, lounging at the next table in upholstered chairs. I walk by, and take in the scent of deep, sweet wood. This was not the checkout line at the Super Center Wal-Mart in Bellefontaine, Ohio, or the light fixture aisle at Home Depot. This was not Paris or Milan. This was Dubai, and it was as if I had landed in a Sunday school poster complete with sandals and sheep—minus sheep, plus Armani. I couldn't make any of it fit—not with Bellefontaine, New York, Paris, or Rome.

I was in the Middle East, and a week earlier, even the sound of that phrase had evoked danger, intrigue, perfume, and tents, as I sat in my makeshift garage office, attempting to arrange bank statements and tax memos. I had accepted a job on the Arabian Peninsula, and I was going to do it; I was determined to carry it through, help set up a college of arts and sciences for Emirati women.

But when I put my foot down for that first step into the Middle East, dragging my American Tourister behind me from the tube of the plane, I emerged into light—light flashing across mirrors and chrome, Jaguars ramped up in displays with enormous red bows, and Rolex counters faceted under refractions of neon in front of metallic palm trees lining the horizon. This was the airport, and I was so stunned I could barely adjust the strap of the carry-on that was cutting into my shoulder.

Dislocation. Setting. Landscape. Out of this, we paint our lives. If we aren't writers, perhaps we can try to make it all fit by using some kind of mental balancing act. We can catalog the cultural oddities and collect observations like foreign postcards. But a writer must pull details from the landscape and paint with words, even while emotion chokes her throat.

I had to get used to the props of the scene: sitting in my car, stranded in lines of Mercedes, BMWs, and Porsches, bumper to hood ornament, honking illogically in the gridlock. No one could move, but the silver ornaments sounded anyway, and most faces gazed stonily through the windows. Taxi drivers, men with hoods, women with only eyes showing above squares of black, spoke into tiny microphones. Windows, anonymous blanks, stared back above massive tires on Range Rovers and Prados. Hummers shone red and VWs sparkled chartreuse—surfaces gleamed and beeped under the desert sun.

I tried to make it fit in those first weeks, but one Saturday morning, I could hear the cornfield across the road from my house rattling its November stalks in the wind. I could see buggies positioned along the far end of Wal-Mart's parking lot, horses breathing steam in the air, black leather offering up cinnamon rolls and honey. Inside Wal-Mart's twenty-four-hour operation, savvy, frugal women with no-nonsense aprons pinned over maroon dresses, white net coverings holding in mounds of hair, were making solemn, calculated purchases in an aisle full of plastic. Little girls in tennis shoes and aprons followed, pushing carts. In the garden aisle, men in flat hats with black suspenders over dark blue shirts, inspected jars of plant food. If I had gone farther up to the Amish store, I would pass them again on Route 68, where manure steamed along the asphalt. And I knew that in my little hallway at home in Ohio, my Great Grandma King's black bonnet and shawl were lying silently in her cedar chest.

Now, through a Ramses-sized window in a pink-mirrored tower, I could see the sun glinting off other jewels lining Sheikh Zayed Road, this eight-lane highway, my front yard. I leaned against the back of my red couch and felt the heat of a coffee cup on the palm of my hand. I set it down carefully, each move an effort, and picked up my calligraphy pen. With this pen, I would center and make it beautiful. I made one sweep of black ink on a scrap of paper, seeking comfort, and then I remembered Mildred.

Her pencil cup materialized with no warning out of the smoke in my mind. A dirty desk in Toledo appeared like a prop in my own *A Thousand and One Nights*. Now, with the sheikh's palace in the distance, laid out in symmetrical wedges of petunias, jasmine, and marigolds, like a paint-by-number canvas in the frame of my window, I remembered that day, two years earlier, when Mildred Benson had spilled water from the plastic wrap around the lilies I had brought as an offering. With dimming sight, she pushed her pencil cup into water pooling in the dust on her desk. Frantically, I offered to get paper towels to wipe up the water dripping down her polyester knee. I had found Carolyn Keene, and I wasn't going to let her go—water, dirt, and a crowlike woman of ninety-three, alive in a navy blue synthetic pantsuit, lingering in the back, gray regions of a newspaper office in Toledo, Ohio. I had found Nancy Drew.

The morning my daughter, Brooke, called to say she had read in *Newsweek* that Carolyn Keene still lived in the guise of one Mildred Benson in Toledo, I had wasted no time. With phone in hand, I told myself that anything I got was a prize. If she could talk at all, I'd hoard a syllable, a breath. After all, this was Nancy Drew, my ninth-grade friend, with pearl necklace, sweater sets, old clocks, and bits of paper.

I scribbled a number on the bottom of a student's first draft, my hand shaking over the scattered desk. And then the tip of my finger punched a formula into plastic squares that would connect me with mystery.

"Hello. *Toledo Blade*. This is Jim," an everyday voice answered. He sounded alive.

"A-a-a, hello. My name is Sandy Humble Johnson. I teach at Bowling Green, and I heard that ... that Carolyn Keene, you know, Mildred Benson, works at the Blade. I wondered if she actually saw people or ..."

"You wanna talk to her?"

"You've got to be kidding? I can talk to her?"

"Yeah, I think she's in. Hold on. I'll connect you."

It was something out of a novel. A novel in a novel. I could smell the musty books lined up in our one-room town-hall library. I could hear them talking, the 1940 girls with happy hair and dogs, under the staircase, lost keys, roadsters, and gloves. I was Howard Carter in the Valley of the Kings, peering through a single mud hole.

"Hello." The voice hardly wobbled.

"Mildred—Mildred Benson? I don't believe it. You're Mildred Benson? Carolyn Keene?" I hesitated and then blurted it out. "Nancy Drew?"

"That's right."

"I'm in shock. It's like a dream."

"Yeah, a lot of people say that." For a second, I thought maybe it was a ruse. The guy who answered the phone didn't hesitate to hook me up with Nancy—it was all too easy. Nancy herself, not sounding ninety-three. But I plunged in. Anything was possible.

"I've read all your books, Mildred. I've read every Nancy Drew mystery."

"Well, they weren't all mine, you know. But I started it."

"No, I didn't know that part. I thought you wrote them all, but maybe I could meet you? Is that possible?"

"Well, not tomorrow, but maybe the day after. You busy on Wednesday?"

"I'll be there. Just tell me where. I'm in Bowling Green, so I'll just drive up."

"One o'clock would be okay. I have to get an article out by Wednesday morning. By one, I'll be done."

"The *Blade*? Is that where I come?"

"Yes, just ask for me at the desk."

"Mildred, I'm thrilled. I'll be there. This is a wonder of the world. I'll be there." My hand trembled as I placed the phone back in its cradle. With Howard Carter, then, at that mud hole, I said out loud, "I see wonderful things."

So in my tower, I remembered that day. There she sat, the reality of unreality, the everydayness of fiction, the lilies, the gray facade of the *Toledo Blade* building, the flesh of Carolyn Keene. Mildred had been on an adventure. Her skin had turned to parchment but she wasn't old. I crumbled the wet paper towel in my hand and brushed it again over her bony knee. I was proud to wipe up the flower water.

"So what do you wanna know?" she said, squinting at me over her damp, dirty desk.

"Start at the beginning, Mildred."

"*The Mystery of the Old Clock*—that was it," she began. A will, an antique clock, and a bold young woman takes to the 1930s highway in her blue roadster. She chooses a yellow sunback dress, carries a handbag, and wears gloves. Even as she looks for clues, her perfect, well-meaning father comments with concern, "It would be looking for a needle in a haystack." But his perfect adventurer daughter replies with determination, "I must figure out a way." And so she did, that Nancy Drew.

I picked up my pen again and stroked the ink, wet and perfect, across a scrap of paper. D-U-B-A-I. Like stitching, this movement of my hand. The rhythm of creation. I'd spent hours of my life with the comforting thud of my Bernina's needle, sewing little dresses for Brooke, ties for Dan, blouses for my mother, and a suit for my sister. *Vogue* and *Butterick* pattern books held my attention for whole afternoons at our Jo-Ann Fabrics. My Bernina had gone with me, with the bobbin case and little red tomato cushion bristling pins that poked through my luggage before I reached Dubai. But it was my friend, this piece of machinery that had witnessed days near the window, a red bird flopping against the glass now and then, as I overcast, made French seams, and dreamed of how we would look in our new clothes.

Clothes. A drape and swag, a scarf with rhinestones, a square of black tied on a face, eyes peering out to register the world, a white net cap, strings dangling, covering hair at Wal-Mart, a black Arab ring, an *'egal*, circling a head like Jesus, a flat hat and vest in the soybean field along Route 68. The world moves under cover, hiding, displaying, saying both *come in* and *stay out*. Clothes bend around the shape of our lives.

Dubai is a theme park peopled with robes, a Disney World in wraps, hotels shaped like Goliath sailboats, Herculean waves, and islands dredged up out of the Gulf to mimic palm trees and a map of the world. Dubai simultaneously laughs and beckons the world to come in and stay out. Last month, returning from my early morning walk along the towers, I came across a movie crew setting up in the predawn light. Three huge vans with beams and cameras were being emptied by buff young men around the entry to Bistro 21, a postmodern, French café for the Emirates airline crew who live in the mirrored monster next to me. Food tents with catered food already were assembled for the crew. I'd seen it all before—this professional, slick filming. I stopped a guy lifting big sound boxes out of the van.

"Are you guys making another movie?"

"Commerical. TV commercial." He draped enormous cables over his shoulder. "We like it here, you know, with all the stewardesses. So what do you do?" he asked.

"I teach. I'm a professor at a university for Emirati women."

"What's an Emirati?" He shuffled some papers into a big plastic binder.

"What's an Emirati?" I'd heard it before, this unknowing, but an early morning crew from London making movies on the stage set that is Dubai, shifting papers and setting up food tents, seemed fictional in itself.

"They're the people who own this country."

Now he looked at me. "Oh, the ghosts. So you know them?"

The ghosts. That's what they have become, my students in black with Gucci, their men in white with Armani. *The shadows*, I heard someone call them later. The shadows glitter. The ghosts laugh. Perfume lingers in the streets. *Come in. Stay out.*

In this Las Vegas of the Arab desert, young women look out through a keyhole onto a scene that is at once a stage set and an interactive computer game. All my students, hooked up experts with IBM laptops, own the game but usually can't play the game. At least not openly. Most of them are behind a curtain in which they move about, looking here and there, without someone asking why a maid didn't iron a blouse that morning.

"Miss, we like it," a student said to me last year. "We don't have to worry about looking good underneath. See, we can just roll in when we're tired." Three girls giggled. One swung open her *abayya* to reveal pajamas. "I was going to wear my fluffy slippers too," she guffawed.

Covering is a way to drive through the world with windows blanked out, to hide that extra bulge or unironed blouse, to study the scene in front of you without being studied. An observer in the thicket. A watcher.

Several years ago, bending over a pile of ungraded papers, I looked up at two figures in black who had suddenly, silently, materialized at my desk. "Miss, it's me—Khulood," one of the cylinders said with enthusiasm. I looked closer at the set of almond eyes blinking above a handkerchief of black.

"Khulood?" I choked out. "You're covering?" And to the other cylinder, I practically shouted, "And you, Noora? Why? Why?" I tried not to sound hysterical.

"We thought about it, Miss, and it's better," Noora laughed. She lifted a hand now clad in black opera-length gloves and reached up under her veil to scratch her nose. I had brought these women through Annie Dillard, Walt Whitman, Sylvia Plath, their faces beaming with each new voice. Now I stared in disbelief at the choice they'd made and realized that my reasoning was useless. They covered to create mystery. It was a cosmetic they had decided to apply. *Come in. Stay out.*

This quiet demand to stay out echoes itself in Logan County, Ohio. To pull my old red Toyota around a black clopping buggy on Route 68, to watch its wooden wheels spew up rain from puddles and warm horse manure, was not a tourist event for me. Horses breathing frost in the air tied up to a post in Wal-Mart's parking lot didn't elicit a second look. The cedar chest in my hall still holds a shawl and bonnet of that world, that world of my grandma's. *Stay out. Come in.*

That's where I came in—that metallic mall with Starbucks, Godiva Chocolate, Donna Karan, and wood perfume.

This week, I watched a Pilipino maid lift a computer bag onto a girl's shoulder. The student, emerging from a white stretch limo, adjusted her Gucci sunglasses, swung her scarf again over her head, and sauntered in glittering high heels to the university's glass doors, which opened automatically as she approached. Her robe ruffled in the desert wind, and I smelled again perfume.

I remember the first time I understood the source of these daily encounters with perfume. I'd gone to the home of one of my students, Asma, for *Iftar*, the evening meal breaking fast after a Ramadan day. I was welcomed to the scene with birds, outrageously gorgeous and foreign. Green and red wings fluttered in cages. First-class photography lined the walls. Cabinets, reaching to cathedral-high ceilings, lit up stacks of silver bracelets, daggers, and discs.

Our meal of fish, rice, dates, honey, and lamb, flat bread with hummus, mangoes, papayas carried in by maids, eventually covered the plastic sheet laid over a silk carpet with yellow and red arabesques. Then, with dessert, a kind of custard coated in sugar, spooned into small bowls, we retired to another room, complete with a huge, flat screen TV. Prancing cartoon kids blinked in from Kuwait. This alone would have joggled me, but the episode that followed took me over the top of my cultural adjustment barometer.

During our meal on the carpet, an elderly man had sat hunched on a chair in the vestibule with his walker propped close by. When his food was served by a maid, I wondered, *a grandfather, an uncle?* Green wings flapped near framed photographs of flowers, yellow and purple. We sat. The old man picked rice with his fingers from the plate.

I leaned close to Asma. "Who's that man in the chair?"

"He's been with my family for I don't know how long. He was a pearl diver on my grandpa's boat. A slave then. He lives with us now. Sometimes with Grandma. Sometimes with us. We respect him." I watched his hand bring a fragment of fish to his mouth. Stunned with this revelation, I lifted another spoon of custard to my mouth.

Now in the TV room, all of us lining the wall on fat pillowed couches, Asma's mother, Sareena, spoke to an Indian maid who was carrying a silver pot on a tray. The maid jetted a flame into a coal of the top of this Aladdin-lamp vessel, and a small coal turned red. Smoke gathered, and then another piece of something was laid on top. All came fast, mysteriously toward me, what with the Kuwaiti cartoon, soft Arab chatter, and the old man pearl diver across the room. Sareena gestured for me, her hand a mosaic of copper-colored flowers.

"Asma, what am I supposed to do?"

"Stand up, Miss. My mother wants to perfume you."

Haze gathered over the silver lamp, and I smiled childishly, not understanding what I was to do with this perfume on fire. I adjusted my long brown sweater and stood, attempting to look assured, part of a ceremony for which I knew no rules. Sareena gestured now for me to turn. She lifted the back of my sweater. Inside, she held the smoking lamp and sweet fog eased between the weave. I attempted to look pleasantly confident in my embarrassment, and I turned when she waved her hand. Then she smoked the front of my sweater, fully knowing I would want this. What woman can be without perfume? Asma smiled, and Sareena smiled, never considering not to offer me perfume. Sisters-in-law smiled, and several children moved closer to the cartoon.

"You'll have this for days," Asma assured me. I grinned and sat down, eager to look part of the scene. A tray of bottles, crystal laced with gold, was presented, and Sareena selected a long gold wand from one container. With this, she stroked the arm of my sweater. She lifted my hair in back and moved a wand from another bottle over my neck. Amber liquid hung on the wand, and she pushed it into the hair at my temples and again above each ear.

Then, she eased out of the couch's stuffed pillows and aimed straight for the pearl diver, who sat humped in a couch across the room. The maid followed with the smoking silver lamp. Responding to an alphabet of gestures incomprehensible to me, the old man read the scene and knew to rise. Grabbing his walker for support, ache spreading over his weathered charcoal face, he submitted willingly to this woman lifting his *kandora* in front and moving the lamp under folds. Within three seconds, his robe smoked and fogged. Unlike me, he knew to turn, and Sareena finished his perfuming in a final sweep of the lamp through his robe.

This woody spice, hanging in the air over sidewalks, along souk windows, inside the walls of Dubai, never dissipates because it's gift and ritual. Essential Arabia. It follows in the swag of black *abayyas*, white *kandoras*, in my brown sweater, and in a pearl diver's robe.

I've been on an adventure, Mildred, and I'm still trying to solve a mystery. But I think I have some clues. A moment of perfume with green birds and silver daggers, a flash, registering metallic palms and Rolex watches, a second of petunias, patch of purple, with the sheikh's mango-roofed palace in a window frame. A flit of a woman's white net strings by plastic dishes at Wal-Mart, a puddle on the road, a rattling of brown corn. Inside my great-grandma's chest, the clothes lay quietly—evidence of a woman who sat on a porch outside of West Liberty, Ohio, with five cats, a dog, and her daughter, my grandma. I know because I have a picture. A camera caught it—that day in 1916, a single live moment on the Earth. Mother and daughter dressed up, picked strawberries, milked cows, and breathed, allowing a record of one summer second: clothes wrapping around their flesh arms, dresses spreading out across the porch, aprons ready for work.

Mildred, you knew.

Now is the mystery. And its unraveling.

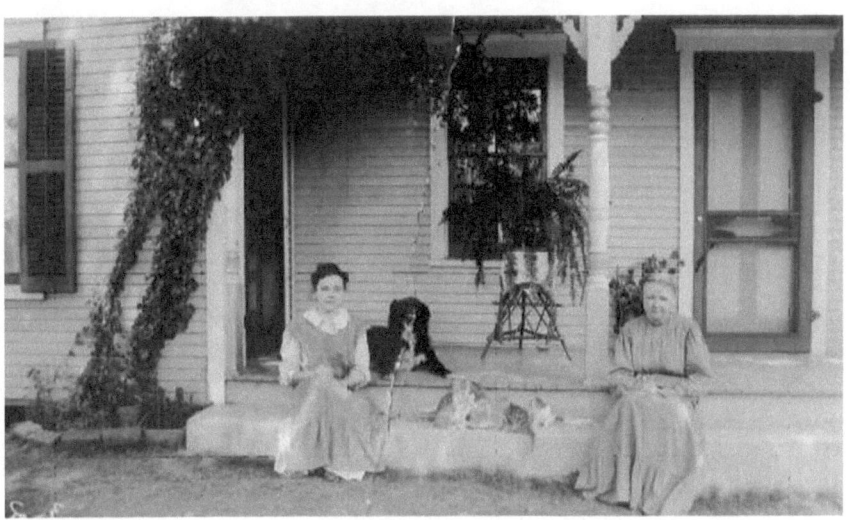

Language

Without knowing it, I knew Elvis would be next on my Christmas mix. I didn't consciously register "Elvis" or click down a mental list of what followed what on the CD Brooke had given me. I heard it. "I-ll-aa-have-aa-a-blue Christmas without you" rang as clearly in my mind as if it were already playing. Johnny Mercer and Margaret Whiting had just finished "Baby, It's Cold Outside" when I heard the King, his thick voice playing off my painted red walls. With December in Dubai, I had played that disc perhaps five times, and five times is all it took to plant a message in my mind—a message without profundity, except that one group of sounds followed another.

This was one more clue about words. If that sound sequence could establish itself in my mind within several weeks, then all repeated patterns could run rivers through my thoughts, dredging the ground deeper with each hearing.

"What is *hadda*, Fatma?" I asked the girl, tying the strings on the back of her veil.

"What, Miss?" Her hands finished twisting the black fabric into a familiar bow over her *shaila*, her scarf, and so I watched her eyes.

"*Hadda*. What is *hadda*?" The eyes looked at two unveiled students sitting in the room with us. Gathering papers and stuffing them into the pockets of IBM bags after class, they ejected sounds between themselves—with courtesy—trying to find out what I was mispronouncing.

"*Had-da*," I offered again.

"Oooh—*hadtha*. Yes, Miss, *this is* my sister. *This is* Miss Sandy. *This is* Kuwait."

"*Hadtha* is *this is*?" And so these sounds had assembled themselves without effort. "Hadtha" was not something these girls thought of consciously. It was already in the program. It was a noise tool. Like a key on the computer. Languages in Dubai are implements for using the day. Pakistani taxi drivers, Emirati women behind the desk at DEWA (Dubai Electricity and Water Authority), Pilipino women behind the checkout counter at Spinneys—all click in and out of languages without effort. They are not thinking. They are not trying. The program changes, and they adapt. William James, the father of psychology, said that habit is a pattern that saves us from tiring.[1] Habit is what we do effortlessly in order to apply the next layer of learning. If a taxi driver had to listen, translate, and strain to form sounds as he adjusted from one language to another, he could not drive his yellow cab through the bumper-to-bumper cars on Sheikh Zayed Road. The checkout girl's "good morning, madam," followed by some stream of rolling sound—gibberish to me—to the bag boy in the yellow shirt beside her, would be impossible. She's Pilipino, and he's Indian, so she's speaking Hindi, or he understands her brand of island talk, or they are speaking some patois that is perhaps a blend of both, plus Arabic. Dubai talk. In and out of sounds without effort. The checkout girl and the bag boy are quick, smiling. For them, language is unconscious.

The goal, then, is to track and dredge what we want. Steer our thoughts back to that painted villa in Rome, that stone farmhouse in Provence, that timber-clad home in Cyprus, and not only will this mind-picture be internally auditory and visual, it will also create a mosaic in time. Thought creates.

Freeman Dyson, the respected British American theoretical physicist, writes about theories of cosmology, which are ever changing. The world built on metaphor and imagination is what he notes, indicating that he is one who would keep the unknown, the unimagined or about to be imagined ideas, that gird up physics. Going beyond "string theory," which is basically the theory of everything (all entities, sounds, chairs, and atoms are waves of energy or "strings" of movement), Dyson leaves the whole scientific world open to the unknown, wisely commenting that "science is inexhaustible."2 Thoughts are waves, created by words—auditory or black marks on paper—and these waves generate physical energy waves in our lives. They bring thought to form. Dyson was right. We don't know how it works. But I see that we create reality. Every minute. Each second. Therefore, I create mine full, balanced, and properly weighted. I create me.

I remember myself always trying. If I could read the right material, join the wisest group, or discipline myself through several days of a new plan, then the whole thing would kick in. I would at last know the secret. I would be trim, wearing those Bermuda shorts my mother made for me in the sixth grade, pulling on that slim skirt without the bulge through my thighs in high school and, when I was married, sewing up *Vogue* patterns without increasing the seams through the hips on a Calvin Klein or Donna Karan. I never gave up.

But I got tired. Sick and tired of trying again and again. Still, I did it. I started over when my disgust winnowed down to a seed of logic. *This is my life*, I said. I must try again, because I refuse to spend the remainder of my years without an attempt, without the pleasure of turning to a mirror, elegant, graceful, and wise, or exploring my Ohio woods in nifty knickers (I pictured myself as an adventurer) or pedaling my new red Schwinn up a hill without giving in to walk it before I reached the top, or selecting Size B panty hose at Krogers. I would not *not* try.

The scenes, though, between those tries are haunting. In one, I'm waiting for my husband, Dan, to come home from work. Lying on the bed with an empty bag of potato chips, a mostly empty bag of Cheetos, and one lone Little Debbie Swiss cake roll in a box next to my head, I can barely breathe or turn over or do anything but wish I wasn't so full. If my stomach hadn't been stretched out like a balloon, I would have taken another frantic bite—to forget, with a momentary taste in my mouth. But I am flat-out on the bed, unable to even look at a Little Debbie, let alone unwrap it. So, for the first few minutes, I breathe and feel sick. Then I think of rattling gravel, telling me Dan is home, and soon he'll tell me everything is all right. And with this thought, comes the eventual hard-breathing resolve that I will not find myself in this bloated position again, disgusted with food that doesn't even do the trick—the trick of covering unwanted feelings, fear, jealousy, fatigue, and confusion. I would find a new plan. That misery on the bed had not allowed forgetting beyond the moment of stuffing.

But why did I do it again? In fifth grade, the other kids offered me their meat relish sandwiches in the cafeteria and, though embarrassed, I said yes. I loved that fresh bread cut in triangles on my plastic, partitioned tray. And then I remember college with the short-lived pleasure of five candy bars on my bunk before some wretched test. And, later, as a teacher, the trigger was three o'clock. That number registered "escape," *get me out of here, I need food right now with Ann and Eleanor,* (They too had been on the front-line, all day teaching), *I need blabbing,* or *I need a piece of sugar cream pie and two dips, no maybe three, of vanilla ice cream.*

A kind of combination panic-denial is the best description I can give of those flailing emotions—something between letting go, not denying myself, and punishing myself for not doing more. And habit. The habit of letting go into chaos. As I looked closely at my own interior, I saw chaos as a way of temporarily resting. If I had chaos, then I didn't have to think; I only had to unwrap the next Snickers and jam its happy chocolate edge into my mouth. Ah, the pleasure of sweetness. And after sweetness, saltiness, with sour cream and onion Pringles. And sweetness again with Bounty or Milky Way. Chaos provides brief comfort, forgetting, and, strangely enough, a launching pad from which to start over again.

Starting over. The clean slate was a comfort too. *See, you did it again, and you're miserable, and you can't take another bite. So you must, you must start over and you will, by the hard breathing of your miserable moment on this bed, find a program and stick to it*—this was my thought process. And this fresh beginning was a salve. But only until approximately three days later, when the system broke down again from desire for that one bite, or that don't-care attitude after school, or that momentary tension with a student. Anything could set me off: ordinary tensions that most people feel but, in my case, emotions that would have to be medicated by jamming something into my mouth.

So, disgust again.

New program. Clean slate.

One bite.

Disgust.

Etc.

I actually did lose weight twice during those years, reaching a goal I had set for myself in a program. I remember the meetings, the euphoria as I neared my target weight number. The striving and the looser clothes. All of it. But those two journeys downward were quickly followed by journeys upward, and no disgust outranked the horror of putting it all back on, with my own fork-hand, after struggling for months physically, psychologically, and spiritually to take it off.

The change that occurred in me nineteen years ago, allowing me to take that journey again and to remain where I wanted to be, came with a shift in words—words I repeated to myself, out loud and silently. And even in their silence, these entities restructured my mind. And mind was what I was trying to fill up.

I painted a scene behind my eyes. First, I made a path, winding through a woods. I was on this path. Sometimes, I would wander to the right to look at a jack-in-the pulpit near the base of a tree. Sometimes, I moved off to the left, to scratch in the leaves for a sponge-top mushroom near a crumbling stump. But right or left, I came back to the path. I didn't scream and flail through the brush, shouting that I must return to my entrance into the woods. I simply found the path again, perhaps a few feet up the way, and I tramped forward.

This path-woods scene replaced an image I had carried for years—the lightbulb. "Lights on" meant I was on the program. One bite of potato salad at three in the afternoon, and it was "lights off." And, although this was a mixed-metaphor shift to paths from lights, it worked for me.

The light switch metaphor represented a border, a clear right and wrong, a good and bad, and, most of all, perfection and imperfection. When I was "imperfect," the light went off, and then I could do two things. First, I could give in to immediate satisfaction and soothing and grab a giant Reeses Cup and bag of M&M's at a gas station I was passing or, at home, rip from the refrigerator the first dangerous bite of unassuming potato salad. Secondly, I could punish myself for not being perfect when I took that first bite of something, somewhere. Even thoughts of bites were punishable by binge.

So, that rigid boundary between two worlds, a line in the sand, a not turning back, an off-and-on light, was the metaphor I replaced with the path. And this replacement, of course, was not only practical in application and result, but also reasonable. In fact, it was more than reasonable; it was a truth of life. Nothing is just one way. We are humans with growth and variation in mood, physicality, desires, and needs. Of course, nothing is just one way—off or on. We are moving up the path. We don't have to start again; we simply have to move back to the center and allow that one forkful from the refrigerator or one bite of a candy bar or one thought of pulling off at Hardee's. It's okay. Back to the path. Moving.

With this scene in my mind, I accepted week by week, and then month into month, a new way of being. I did not panic or punish. I saw myself returning to the path, a human being, acting in a wise way. Words and pictures. Pictures and words. Language creates. Words turn gold and rest behind eyes. Elvis sings without thought, and I walk forward in my slim skirt.

Tents and Inspector Gadget

The advent of my arrival in Dubai was heralded, hauntingly, by tents and Inspector Gadget. On the day I broke with my university in Ohio, because I didn't receive the position I believed should have been mine, the day I cut the cord and said, "You are done, Sandy," I wandered, stunned and half-numb, down the diminutive street that backed onto my smaller-than-diminutive apartment.

Down the alley that was called a street, I walked, into the room that was advertised as an apartment, I entered, and onto the foam rubber that was named a bed, I flung my red turtleneck, red leather gloves, red winter scarf, and red beret. Tomorrow I would tell them. But tonight, I would cry. The foam rubber futon Brooke and I had bought together covered most of the apartment's floor. Here, I sprawled in the bumps and pillows. Here I sobbed, tired, running my hands over the cockeyed foam, the rough green cover. The yellow pillowcase received my calligraphic smears of mascara as I bellowed and coughed.

At last, when I turned over, I looked up into the Martha Stewart curtain I'd found at Kmart. One end of it hung over a huge branch Dan had cut for me, ten years before. Up the side of the dirty, pocked plaster wall rose a cardboard tree and, dangling from several of its one-dimensional branches, crystals. Crystals. Tacked, nailed, at the tips of brown paper twigs. Old wood branch. Fake tree. Shimmering glass. Gauzy curtain.

When I first concocted this collage, I thought *a combination of Thoreau's cabin and a Bedouin tent. Yes, that's it.* Out of the wild of my life. Out of the words of my mind—the traveling house, the portable hearth, the something out of nothing. That was what I was trying to do. With Thoreau, I wanted "a house which you have gotten into when you have opened the outside door, and the ceremony is over ... such a shelter as you would be glad to reach in a tempestuous night, containing all the essentials of a house ... where you can see all the treasures of the house at one view, and everything hangs upon its peg."[3]

Because Brooke had not been able to tolerate university life and had gone back home to West Liberty, we had taken on a reversal of roles: daughter in home, mother in college apartment. So I used all the plastic apartment-setup paraphernalia she had left behind—a blue and yellow mix-and-match set of dishes from Wal-Mart, a periwinkle dish drainer, and blue and yellow towels. And the cheap futon where I lay, staring into the Martha Stewart drape.

I thought about the eight months in this one room. I had happily brewed up lentils and beans, used old asparagus cans for pencil holders, and operated a secondhand microwave I'd bought for ten dollars at a yard sale from some graduating senior guys who found themselves with five ovens at the end of four years. At Goodwill, I picked up three nesting baskets for fifty cents and a comforter with an impressionistic tree painted on its fabric front. Something from nothing.

Now lying there, looking up into my halfway tent, I realized, dully, that this letting go was both less and more than my last university exit. This university, my doctoral school, was a state school. It didn't have the last university's airs, parading as the Harvard of the Midwest. *Pompous journal-writing bores*, I thought, shifting on the futon, its response a brash, spongy return to its original bulge. But this university, my school—here, I had been one of the people I knew, one of the commoners, an Ohioan, helping young men and women. Ohio kids, Midwestern kids. I knew it sounded sentimental, missionaryish, but this teaching was something out of nothing too.

I stood up, rubbed my cloudy contacts, picked up the phone, and punched in numbers.

"Diana?"

Our conversation carried forward in fits and starts as I laid the event out before my friend.

"So, Sandy, your degree is in English literature?" the man said.

"Nineteenth-century British, you see, because I wanted Wordsworth. Because I wanted the spots of time."

"Ah, 'The Prelude.'" I felt a jab. The man knew my territory, my knowledge of the poet's epic. I didn't want anyone to take it away from me.

I'd been ragged and shocked for three weeks, settling my emotions this Sunday morning by insisting on the full collection of Inspector Gadget parts from the local McDonald's. With a styrofoam cup in each hand, swishing brown vicious coffee, I'd made my way to Diana's. On the table lay an assemblage of Gadget's arms, legs, and head spinning helicopter blades. Shifting a plastic pouch with Gadget's combo torso and clock, I decided that it was good to have someone know enough to respond to the great cache of knowledge I jealously guarded.

"But what about you, Abe? This thing in the Middle East. What an adventure. What is it? Tell me."

The man in Bermuda shorts laughed easily. "It's an adventure, alright. You know, Elaine and I spent five years in Cairo. And I guess when this thing appeared in the *Chronicle*, I knew I didn't really want to retire. I just took it up, and here I am. On my way to gather a faculty for a new university—actually it opened last year—but new."

"Where? Arabia, Diana said."

"Dubai."

"Dubai?" I didn't know the name.

"That's the city. The country—tiny, oil, rich—the United Arab Emirates."

An intense, circling bird, Diana perched on the chair next to me. "Tell her about the life of these Arabs, Abe."

"Well, this is not a bunch of tents and camels." Abe motioned to his wife to take a chair. "You want a cup of coffee, Hon?" I hadn't noticed his accent before. French? Greek? I couldn't place it.

Elaine finally sat on the other side of the table, tapping her cup, eyeing her husband. "Cairo—I'll miss Egypt. But this will do—the Middle East. Not the craziness of the markets, like the last five years. But Abe thinks he always has to move on, you know. He thinks he's got to do this thing."

"Sounds glorious. Adventure. What's the whole thing about, anyway, but adventure?" I guessed they were in their sixties, and here they were on their way to Arabia, sophisticated in taking a chance, playing it big.

During the past year, before May, even before the current event, I'd toyed with another continent. A move. The Second Language program. For one night, I had tried to live in the same house as the head of that department—Anita Duke—who had on that one night suggested China.

"You know, Wes Longman and Pat spent last year there and loved it. You could try it, Sandy," Anita had said. "They respect their professors." But although the language program, TESL, was laudatory, I considered it something less than my mystical union with words, letters, and poetry. No, I couldn't go with an organization that identified itself with an acronym. I opted out.

"Dubai. Towers growing out of the desert. Wealth. Mercedes, Jaguars, cars. These Arabs have wealth. And I respect them for wanting to educate their women," Abe was saying as I tuned in.

"You've been there, Abe?"

"When we were in Egypt—I think in ninety-three—or, Hon, was it ninety-four?"

"Ninety-three," Elaine Kyrie offered, her mind a repository of their travels.

"And then three weeks ago, I accepted the job. Dean. We'll put together a college of arts and sciences. It's incredible. The architecture in Dubai. Money to throw away. And this university has the potential for growth. To be on the ground floor in forming a university—that's the opportunity. Quite frankly, I couldn't turn it down."

"I always wanted to start a university. Something little. With the right ingredients—just a few buildings. With experts in each discipline. And then just let them carry on. Doing what they do." I stood one Gadget leg up on the table and took another swig of coffee.

Jake, a colleague and friend, and I had toyed around with a plan for a university during the past five years. "Dr. Griffith," I would address him, and he would return with "yes, Dr. Johnson?"

"Let's start a university. The right way. Get rid of this academic mumbo-jumbo. It's a labyrinth of form that kills us and kills the students. It's got to be possible to be free and learn."

"Yeah, I've thought of it. Many times. But how? How do you start without funding? Without the involvement of these bastards?" We'd wander off then, Jake and I, fantasizing about the hillside where we'd build the first structure in our university.

"So, why don't you apply?" Diana was leaning down now, straightening a reed mat in the middle of the table.

"What?" I pulled back from thoughts of my Ohio hill university to this kitchen, this offer.

"Why not apply? Sandy may be just what you need in Dubai, Abe." Diana was using her no-nonsense, mother tone.

"Well, why not? Think about it, Sandy."

"I wrote a book, you know. I'm proud of it."

"That's great. What subject?"

"Time. You know the spots of time in 'The Prelude'?"

"Of course. So why not Arabia?"

"Why not?" The ridiculous possibility of it suited me. "What would you like to see—resume? Book? What?"

"Send your credentials, and when we get back from California, I'll take a look at them."

Incredible. Absurd. A dream. I scooted all my Gadget parts into the white Happy Meal bag. "I'll do it, Abe. This might be the time. Dubai."

Down the alley that was called a street, I walked, into the room that was advertised as an apartment, I entered, and onto the foam rubber that was named a bed, I dropped my bag of Inspector Gadget parts. I stood on my toes, stretched up into the folds of my Kmart tent, and lifted the first crystal leaf off its cardboard tree.

On the screen, Inspector Gadget's hat twirled. Copter blades lifted him up between buildings. Lighting again on the sidewalk, he sprung awkwardly, ajar, from his right shoe. My fingers itched, hot and greasy, but I dipped again into the box, mechanically, not able to resist the magnetism of popcorn.

"Miss, do you like it?" In the flitting light of the screen, I could see an outline of black, round flesh between, eyebrows arched, red-purple lips. The smell of wood perfume.

"It's … it's … interesting. In a kind of cartoon—" My whispering, popcorn-filled mouth lost itself in a flare of clapping, shouts over the red plush. "You see, before I came, I bought this Inspector Gad—" But the draped head was entirely black now, the student having leaned away to the other side. A roar raged over my explanation, my light telling, this cartoon gone mad.

Whenever I had tried words on this feeling behind my breast, I thought *ache, tight, dull*. I kept it in, lurching from episode to episode, but when I was too worn out to fit it neatly into some pattern to put away in my mind, a base from which to work, when I stopped, cold, dead in my mental tracks and remained passive—it's then I collapsed behind my eyes. Active. Passive. The active pattern had pushed me to say, "Yes, I'll chaperone. What do I do?" The passive pattern held me in the seat of the Galleria Cineplex with my mouth open like a fish, sucking in popcorn. The movie was *Inspector Gadget*. And the little plastic man, who looked the same as the one riding the plastic screen in front, confronting the world ineptly, heroically, bungling ahead with Don Adams's voice, sat on a back shelf in my garage. Ohio.

The Cave

Impermanence, mutability, mold in the refrigerator, clothes scattered from the night before—all these could initiate cave time.

The cave was a dark mood, the sight of my own flaws. Here I darkened and wanted to run away. Here I darkened and wanted to cover myself. Here I darkened and wanted to eat. The cave was malaise, ennui, and the inability to desire a walk or muster the strength to uncover a head of lettuce. The inability to move. The cave was recognition of mortality and imperfection, and imperfection wanted to become perfect, and perfection was impossible. But with language, I could make my way and change the metaphor. And just as my path needed to wander forward through Ohio woods, my cave also needed an exit. It would, in fact, not be a cave, but a brief transit through a tunnel, and this tunnel would have a light at the end.

I had heard someone say, "Just feel the feeling,"—even if it was despair, jealously, or boredom, and my initial response had been "but I need to be active in my search to do it all right, even as I move along the path." The cave, however, held me, with little energy to get up on the path again. While the path indicated motion and the ability to do something, an action, the cave indicated just sitting there passively. So I decided to try "feeling the feeling"—the whole smear of life's disappointments and guilt—without the medication of food. And with that decision, I made a plan to prepare myself for the cave by setting up a list of things I could do as I sat in darkness or passed through the tunnel: eat lettuce that was already shredded, open a can of green beans, walk, talk to someone, drink water. The cave would reveal itself as a tunnel if I waited it out with small alterations to my activities, little acts. I blabbed to my friends, I ate green beans, and the mood passed.

Moods shift. Richard Carlson taught me years ago in his book *You Can Be Happy No Matter What*, that you can wait out a damaging emotion and that you will come out on the other side.[4] The Dalai Lama suggests, in the same vein, that we need to "play turtle" and pull back until a destructive emotion passes.[5] I would add to Carlson's and to the Dalai Lama's comments that the waiting feels messy and uncontrolled, and that's what you have to be ready for—the messiness of emotion.

Earlier, when I placed myself in a "program," I'd say, "This time, absolutely, I'm doing it. Nothing can make me take that bite." But then the cave would appear with its own policies, its own ether, its own government, which eventually resolved into the anarchy of *who cares anyway? Life is short. I need potato chips. I'm going to die, so why can't I have a piece of cheesecake, lingering there on the second shelf of my refrigerator? Just like everyone else. I need it.* But by knowing that my cave had an opening, I sat in the darkness, felt the imperfection of those excuses, and told myself *You will come out on the other side. Just wait. A few minutes, maybe hours, but you will see a light. Do something. Something not damaging.* Hence, the water, the beans, the lettuce, the walk, the talk. My list was composed of items that filled me, and that was what I needed. Not only did these activities give the sensation of filling me, but they actually aided in my weight loss. Water was cleansing. Lettuce and green beans supplied vitamins and growth. Walk involved moving my muscles. Talk allowed me to link up with other human beings and learn from empathy, sympathy, giving, and taking.

I did come out the other side. As sure as morning passed into afternoon, a light appeared at the other end. The light was inevitable, if I just waited and felt the feeling. Simple and yet profound. In the light, looking back, I applauded myself for enduring, for eating that huge salad when I wanted a Dunkin' Donut, and for laughing with a friend when I wanted to "be like everyone else" and wallow in food, alone. I learned that darkness comes to all of us but will dissolve with time. I found this in Ohio and carried it to Dubai.

Red Couches and Refrigerator

"The red."

"Certainly, Madam. A brilliant color. And you'd like two?"

"Yeah, let's go all the way. Two couches in red. In the desert. For some reason, even in this heat, I need red. Is that weird?" I realized then that Elmo, the Pilipino decorator at IKEA, probably could care less if the couch was green, pink, or purple; he would sidle up to any buyer. On the other hand, I reasoned, he must be involved with color. Maybe color gave him life.

"Madam, red is important, bold. It must be red for you."

"Thank you, Elmo."

I fumbled with the sheets of paper I'd come to know as money—the *dirham*. Five hundred with a falcon head and mosque, one hundred with more falcons, and ten with a bird again, a date palm, and a *khanjar*, which is a vicious-looking dagger. Even this wadded paper kept me plunging back and forth in my mind, adjusting, and the walk I'd made earlier down the middle of City Center Mall had drained away almost everything I had in my emotional balancing store. *Calm, remain calm*, I told myself.

Now, as I watched Elmo click my payment into the computer, I braced myself to go out again under the mammoth tent canopy, to be followed by the smell of something I didn't recognize. Spices? Perfume? Chicken? Whatever it was, it was always there, drifting between Donna Karan, Ralph Lauren, and the rows of gold shops.

"You'll deliver?"

"Of course. Your address?"

"I'm not sure. You see, there's no street number. I live in a pink, mirrored tower." No other way to describe the situation emerged from my vocabulary. Along with robes and desert-wide mobile phones had come twelve-lane highways, lined in glittering towers with no numbers. But Elmo didn't miss a beat. This absurdity did not move him.

"And the name of the tower?"

"Oasis."

"The flat number?"

Scrambling again for a foothold in symbols, such as numbers, letters, or anything to place myself down on the new road in the new box of my apartment, to tell this confident face that didn't care about my green hill in Ohio, I blurted out, with strained buoyancy, "Twelve-zero-seven." Elmo punched at his keyboard, and the deal was done.

That had been yesterday, my second Thursday in the Emirates, the Arab Saturday. I had lined up delivery dates, furniture, plates, forks, and spoons at IKEA, but my strength had ebbed. My will had weakened. Two weeks of buying, glamorous and meaningless, churned up conflict, searing, and constant. I could buy but could not attach emotion to these objects. This was the Peace Corps with glitz. An adventure created by the gods. On the edge of fear and delight. Nothing could have been more suited to my nature, but I was worn. And afraid. Not of the Emirates, exactly. But something behind my ribs.

Now I wrapped my fingers more tightly around the carriers topping my IKEA bag—even the wrappings were flashy. I had etched out today's plan. After groceries at Continent, I would return the silverware. I preferred clear handles rather than dark red. But since Friday was "Sunday," I had to jam everything into store openings after two. Coordinating. Exquisite coordination of my life. I propped a half-smile on my face, determined to walk tall in my black suit—the one I'd made fifteen years earlier for a trip to New York. But behind the black lapels of my Calvin Klein, I hurt.

On the other side of a huge, grated metal door, I could see workers in yellow shirts scrambling to rearrange piles of shoes and pyramids of mangoes. Five minutes to go before the grate would ease up, receiving a flood of black robes, white robes, red checked scarves, carts with dangling children, and me. Now I waited, looking up again at windows lined in gold bracelets, bigger gold necklaces, flashing signs, crystal bottles, and diamonds. Perfume and spice coated my throat. I had to sit down. So I did—right on the marble floor, my back leaning against the edge of a pharmacy with Nokia displays. I looked at my watch—1:57. Waiting. My life. A flock of *abayyed* women glanced at me and smiled. I heard soft Arab chatter.

But then I was up again to secure a cart. I refused to think the word "trolley." It irritated me. It was British, not American. "I'll get a cart and smile and wait the minutes," I said in my own language to my wounds.

Standing, I leaned against the wall, the cart in front, the mask in place. Suddenly, two women of the flock were there, making sounds, gesturing at my pants.

"What?"

They pointed again at my Calvin Kleins and, even though they smiled, I feared I had made some mistake, some cultural faux pas. They touched my jacket. I turned. White dust imprinted the marble wall down my left leg, and chalk outlined the pharmacy window up my left arm.

"Oh, thank you. I see. I see." What sweetness, I wanted to say, but could only repeat my gratitude with volume. My loud words made no sense.

Language—where it keeps us and where it takes us—was another lesson. An unknown language, the bearer of compassion, lifted, if only for a moment, my displacement, my overwhelming knowledge that things bring brief satisfaction, my nagging fear of nothingness. The metal grating creaked, an opening appeared, and we leaned forward on our carts, into the shoes and mangoes.

Some moments I felt outside of time's sweep, full in a circle of activity, attention focused on what I wanted to do. But on other days, I saw it all rushing, running ahead me, and for hours, I could not get back. Morning, noon, and evening clogged with time-things, reminders of life's forward swing.

I glanced, reluctant, at the table. Papers lay cockeyed and threatening, peppered with yellow Post-it notes, waiting for a hand to shift them into a master plan for the college of arts and sciences we were creating. Unsymmetrical and needy, the piles longed for attention and order. And my hill in Logan County rose far beyond this beige drift of sand. Brooke, gray fur kneaded under her fingers, would be sitting on the couch with Kitty. Now these odd-sized strangers, these A-4 papers, were not allowing me to inhabit my circle. They were sentinels of Dubai acts, tedious, hot, and tiring, and I acknowledged that most life lay outside the circle.

But just as I reached out to subdue an A-4, I remembered Christmas. Christmas in Dubai, of course, and lights. This was the city of lights and mirrors. And water. The Creek. I had heard of dinner served in the mahogany-colored dowels docked up on the salt-water inlet from the Gulf. Drifting among the vertical electricity of towers, rocking under the moon in the dark air—*that is it*, I thought. *I will spend Christmas on the Creek.*

I wanted to tell someone. I wanted to arrange this composition with words. This gilt-edged event was a staged moment, replete with Arab mystery and Ohio memories. Under a Dubai moon, I would still be able to picture Willie Yoder, rubber-banded into his white beard, propped in a sleigh on a wagon pulled by a John Deere down Main Street. Kids would breathe frost along the sidewalks while "ho, ho" blasted from speakers perched up the light poles, punctuating the four corners of our one-street downtown. And I, easing up the Creek, would rock in a boat, scanning the navy blue waters of an Arabian inlet.

It sounded dangerous and romantic, like the scheme of a nineteenth-century explorer, and so I honed it, this scene. My friend David would listen. Even from San Francisco. He would like my painting of words, water, and lights.

When he didn't answer, I flopped into my rattan chair, disappointed, watching the sun rage up orange over a smear of foggy water in the distance. I needed to talk.

But with one more breath in and out, I picked up my pen, walked to the refrigerator, and took down a half-sheet of A-4 tucked under a magnet. I tore the paper in half, opened the door under the sink, and threw it in. I opened the laminated menu I used for a desk and took out one clean, full sheet. This I folded and tore in half, laying one piece on the top of the makeshift menu desk and the other on the marble counter to the side of the burners. Uncapping my Shaeffer, I eyed the nib—medium, my favorite—and touched down on the torn edge with my code. *Pro Fat Milk Brd Fruit*, I swept across the foreign A-4 in black calligraphy. I capped the pen, laid it diagonally on the menu, to the top right of the subdued paper, and opened the refrigerator door. This ceremony of ink and food steadied my day.

But with the refrigerator door open, releasing blank cold breath from a white mouth, I teetered. I told myself it didn't have to be a dark, Earth-wobbling act to look at these shelves. It was the way of the world—foodstuff, growing white edges programmed to turn green. Food that smelled sour when I unscrewed a plastic lid. *No, this is diurnal*, I whispered inside my head; it is rhythmic, a song, an evolution of grass, fiber, and kin. But the shelves, shifting this way and that, with jars of mayonnaise and relish, a bottle half-full of V-8, and a plastic skin covering Louis Rich turkey bacon, represented vast plans that had passed, dwindled, or hadn't happened at all. They had been luxury liners, ships pulling out of port, engineered celebrations. But now what strategy of dishes and oven timer these suspicious crusts of green scorned. Circles of delicate red and lime laughed up from under a plastic lid when I uncovered the potato-broccoli casserole from the week before. Mold reminded me, like Ozymandias's ghost returning. I cringed in the dull cold of the refrigerator's passive white face. Look on my works, ye mortals, and despair.

I shut the door with a thud, opened the freezer, checked the Lean Cuisine cannelloni's protein and carbohydrates, slid it back in the cold, and scrolled my formula on the torn A-4. Whatever happened, I would be trim. I would slip the narrow skirt over my hips. Back to the path.

Small Slices

All life proceeds in small slices—moments, one at a time. Thus, it's reasonable to conclude that all life alterations must also proceed one small piece at a time. This I learned by acting first and observing later. Acting first meant moving without thinking—that is, without a thinking that dissects, questions, pulls back, and disassembles. Instead I thought ahead. I laid out a plan and understood in this plan there would come some "cave" moments. All I had to make was one small slice—one exercise, one pinning up of my half-sheet of paper, one glass of water, one less step with a spoon toward the casserole, one, one, one, one.

Yes, catastrophic moments occur, shifting our lives dramatically; however, changes of habit, even after life-altering single events, must still move us forward. Since I had this logic before me and desired this change, I did one step—the first of a thousand miles—to get me there. It worked. It works. So then, when I was losing weight, and now, as I maintain my body, I act first and feel later. The act itself becomes a joy, a completion. I relax in a single slice.

Recent experiments on the brain by prominent neurosurgeons, psychiatrists, and other thinkers in this area have shown that the pathways in the brain alter with small steps. I'm not a scientist, but my own life, viewed through the lens of logic, suggests to me that any change of behavior or thought must necessarily be physically shaping pathways in that area behind my eyes. I was willing, early on, to simply make verbal adjustments without verification of this physical fact, which is evident now through scanners, sound waves, and computer technology. But I'm gratified to learn that what I seized at in the dark is currently a positive finding and a focus of physicians. The brain can be restructured.

The new field of cognitive neuroscience, revealing specific motions in the brain, goes beyond tenets of behavior and cognitive psychology. At the head of this study is Richard J. Davidson, director of the Laboratory for Affective Neuroscience at the University of Wisconsin-Madison, who has verified links between the brain and the emotions that shape neurological pathways. The brain, in fact, has a plasticity that allows it to change throughout an individual's life. New neurons are created that connect areas of the brain, which then alter our emotional lives. Davidson reports that "new neurons do grow through the entire life span."[6] This information validates what happens when we change words that track through our minds. We say the words, we see the image, and then we make new paths. Literally, then, the path in my metaphor, where I return to the center rather than going back to the beginning of my journey, is a neurological road through the labyrinth of my mind.

This knowledge is power. It's small and large at the same time. That is, it gives us the okay sign to do something we can do. We can all handle one motion toward a project. One stitch. One thought. Do and think—and think only the can-do-it thought. Yes, all the old positive reinforcement clatter is not clatter. It's the way. It's the single way, the small slice that shapes our brains and bodies.

Facade and Faux

University life in Dubai was not crumbling stones with ivy. Not like Oxford, England, or Oxford, Ohio. Not even like my state school, Bowling Green, with its unmatched buildings, where an attempt to shape structures into creatures or objects had made the gym into a brick falcon. Even there, I had enjoyed the mystery of knowledge clashing, layer upon layer; even there, I had found places in which I could forage and discover something hidden, an abandoned black shutter from a nineteenth-century house, back in an alley; a crumpled note, tucked in the pages of a library book; a cardboard Elvis, smirking from the corner of the pop culture library. Layers allowed discovery. Around the corner. Just ahead. There, Schleimann uncovered Troy, and Carter dug up Tut. It was the waiting, the loneliness on the sand for a decade, the accidental shovel load of desert that scuffed the first descending step, a hole in a mud wall that allowed the words "I see wonderful things."

Searching spun energy. Mystery was essential.

But corners were squared and lines straight in Dubai. At least on the surface. The sun glared down on walls in rectangles, and the system was to be cleaned and lined up, and, in its symmetry, the best. The Arabs of Dubai insisted on the pinnacle. To build higher. To create a surface shinier than the shiniest object on the globe. This better-than preoccupation not only included gold-leafed Rolls Royces, but handbook presentations created by the latest Photoshop program, offered up with the glossiest covers. Plastic inside plastic, faux leather, and lists of content in multiple fonts. Inside pockets. Outside pockets. Facade.

And I believed in facade. I planned and calculated for years various scenarios, even once in tenth grade, wearing a hot brown wool suit, my thinnest outfit, in the middle of a July day, so that Jim Greer would spot me out his window as I strolled casually, ridiculously, to the ballpark. What was my body but a cover I maintained for presentation of entry into a room, all dressed up for opening the lone glass door at Dajolee's, West Liberty's one restaurant? A walking art form. What went with me, perfumed and arranged.

But the Arabs of Dubai had outdone me in this matter of presentation. It seemed to me that, in their culture, facade was center; that is, the surface came first, a gleaming exterior. And when I thought about it—why not? Maybe I had it all backward, by putting this search for the soul first. This interior construction. Perhaps we should all build facade first, whether it is athletic superiority or beauty—our choice. Do the body up front, with clothes, earrings, and muscles, and later fill in the frame with humanity. I witnessed in Dubai exterior preceding interior. Scaling down did not equate to holiness. Any momentary thought of a sackcloth-and-ashes approach to life was my blunderbuss-and-big-collared-pilgrim past speaking. And as I recalled the dusty framed print, hanging at the far end of my ninth period study hall in Ohio, I remembered that even those painted Puritans insisted on flair with stiff collars and lace froth at their seventeenth-century necks. We all set a tone, whether we are Massachusetts Pilgrims, me in my July wool suit, or Emirati Arabs. In Dubai, tone involved glamour and prayer.

I thought about it almost every day. And if I wasn't thinking about it at the top of my mind, I was laughing about it, arranging it, and scorning by it on a buried level. But not so buried as it had been in Ohio. In Dubai, it emerged often. It stood right up there as philosophy, a way of being, practical and, most revealing, a part of reality. Faux.

Yes, faux, fake, not the real thing. Like my Wal-Mart diamonds, my zircons. I remember a woman, with her man, in Newark. Several years ago, I'd been passing through that smudged American city, feeling the drama of my Middle Eastern life, standing at a curb to be transferred to JFK, when the man spoke.

"On your bag—what is that? Do you teach at a university? What language is that? Arabic?"

"Yes," I said, pleased that in this tawdry space, my embossed university bag, scrolled in Arabic, faux black leather, hinted at adventure.

These two were kind and interested, so I told the tale, as much as I could narrate in ten minutes. The pink tower, the perfume, the perceived danger, the cars. And then it was there—the longing on their faces. I saw it and understood it. Together, midforties, educated, they were ready for something else.

"And your earrings. Beautiful. Diamonds, right?"

"Wal-Mart."

I loved this part. The rule had become this: when a small, inexpensive item resides in the region of balance and form, the small, cheap thing becomes rich in the mind of the beholder. Those crystals looked good in their setting, the ear, the airport, and the story. I've often questioned why one would save for a lifetime to buy a stone that flashes for a few seconds in a room. Paper and metal, bills and coins, our bartering agents, can better be used to create a larger form, beauty of body, a tilted beret, a college degree. Why would one dangle a rock, suffered for and saved for, when, in the presence of balance, a zircon transmogrifies into a diamond in the mind of the beholder? This is the magic of proximity. The desire of others to have what they think they don't have.

"Really? They look expensive. Like diamonds." But both of us knew, the woman and I, that one thought had followed the other. Middle East wealth. Towers. Arabs. Rolls Royces. Diamonds. And although I enjoyed this on multiple levels, some of which I didn't like to face in myself—*see, I look good with cheap; see, you're impressed with drama; see, your gaze holds steady with this tale of adventure; see, you think you want what I have*—this curbside meeting panned out as philosophy.

"Do they need more teachers?" the woman offered, humbly, hungrily. "I have my masters in clinical psychology and another in sociology."

"Oh, wonderful. What a combination. But—," and here I touched the woman's arm, knowing her taste, understanding that ravenous hunger for change, "what is your name?"

"Angela."

"And yours?" I touched the man's sleeve.

"Paul." He leaned forward, just a fraction.

"Angela, Paul, you could try, but the red tape is unbelievable … papers, visas, and now with the New York thing …"

"Yes. It must be difficult to get around …"

"I don't know what it would take now," I had to admit. "But where are you going?" Three vans now stood in line against the curb, the last having the inscription "Terminal Transfer."

"We … we're going back to Philadelphia." Angela's voice, softer now, seemed embarrassed, as if she were trying to hide that U.S. city.

"Good luck," I said, and I was off. Earrings and mystery, I left them with a whiff of Arabia, concern, danger, and education for world peace. It was the Wal-Mart secret. Faux had it all.

And faux equals form. All form comes to copy something.

Some Thing. Form equals faux. A painter copies a tree or house or hand. A musician copies the sounds of birds and wind, a traffic jam. A writer copies the assembling, careening jumble of mind, behind her eyes.

And Dubai copies Venice.

Before the second *Eid*, *Eid-Al-Fitr*, marking Abraham's substitution of sacrifice, before I saw Venice in its watery flesh, the Mercato mall opened on Jumeirah Beach Road, replete with the Grand Canal painted in its entry. Pink, green, and dusty blue shutters, flanking flower boxes on fake houses, arched over the automatic doors of Dubai's latest amalgamation of Armani, Pachi, Mango, and Missoni. That mall mural solidified my decision to go back to Italy. I picked up the latest Andrea Bocelli CD at Virgin, packed carefully my acrylic furs from Ohio, and I was off on Lufthansa with a reasonable price into Milan and then to Marco Polo, the Venice airport. But after the fantasy of a canal water taxi with Michelangelo, my twenty-six-year-old boatman, after a heavy door opened onto immaculate white sheets and towels, foil-wrapped chocolates, and closets with automatic lights and safe, after the armoire opened easily, elegantly, to reveal a TV, my hand clicking the remote, which bannered a greeting across the screen, "Welcome, Mrs. Johnson," after the shock, once again, of more and more, of excess, there they stood on the flashing glass in my Venetian palace—the Emirates Towers. The screen was advertising the view from my bedroom window in Dubai.

I had come from the desert, thousands of miles, to the cake-frosting glimmer of Venice, to be welcomed by a framed picture of my daily window in Arabia. "Come to Dubai, the city that puts the world on the map."

I shivered in the damp of watery walls, pulled on my furs, tilted my beret, and forced my desires down to the canals, knowing that the world perpetually wants something else and that faux equals form.

There he was—flat straw hat and striped shirt—his boat scrolled in gold, sloshing against the side of a green wall.

"Do you have blankets?" I yelled.

"Signora, come down. Of course, not too cold today."

"I'm freezing. What's your name?"

"Francesco."

"I'm freezing, Francesco, but I have to do this."

He held out his hand, and I stepped into the gondola's shell. Covering me with a brown blanket, he offered his opening line: "Signora, do you want the regular or the Marco Polo tour?"

"Marco Polo, of course."

He dipped his oar into gray green, and we slid forward on light and air.

Full

On some days, I denied what my body knew, and holidays in Ohio provided one of the greatest denials—the meaning of food. Thanksgiving, Christmas, Halloween, Valentine's Day—name a month, and I'll give you a "food day." How could I possibly face those kitchen counters steaming with casseroles in November and deny myself my sister-in-law's broccoli-chicken delight? What about my Aunt Marjory's cherry cheesecake, my Aunt Violet's yeast rolls, or my mother's noodles? What's Thanksgiving for, anyway? Brownies, chocolate chip cookies, fresh, warm. I told myself that, at some level, my body didn't need to register those holiday bonanzas. My body needed to splurge on some days, and those days should not "count" in my program, whatever the program was at the time.

But food near the top of my pleasure list brought chaos. It was lurking there in my mind long before Dan, Brooke, and I pulled into the driveway where cars had been tucked in along the gravel or in the grass near the chicken house. Brothers and sisters-in-law had carried in covered glass dishes and bulging bags. Chaos was waiting in those bundles, because on those particular days, food meant not just eating, but wallowing—in family, in living, in my cultural rights. Those days meant taking as many turns back to the casserole table as I jolly well desired. But just like the moment on the bed with an empty Little Debbie box, this moment of holiday denial sabotaged itself. I could only take so much into my stretched stomach; eventually, I couldn't even muster up the desire to get to the table again, and the logic of coming to this impossibly stuffed stage brought disgust. I'd sit on the couch and laugh, breathe heavily, and laugh some more. But already the feeling of "tomorrow morning" was setting in. Bitter. Why couldn't I laugh, eat, be part of my own life, and not feel miserably heavy and out of control? Wasn't there a way to enjoy life, with much of it including food, and not be crippled by illogical actions?

The quandary generally revolved around a set of ideas: *I must be on my program, moving toward my goal weight. But I'm a human being who needs food anyway, so why can't I have the unmitigated pleasure of just digging in on these holidays and not thinking? I have just eaten enough to feed a normal family of five, and I feel miserable. Can't I have food pleasure and life pleasure too? I must be on my program, moving.*

And so these ideas circled around in my skull as I approached the morning following the holiday. But since most days weren't holidays, I had to face the aftermath of such illogical thought during the bulk of my days, with my thighs spreading out wide on the kitchen chair as I sat down again to think.

The answer eventually resolved itself into an elementary simplicity: My body is with me all the time. If I feed it outrageously at the casserole table, it takes the chicken delight in and all the layers of stuff that follow. My body can't save itself from my food holidays; it's there, preholiday, holiday, and postholiday, and will register its intake with expanded fat cells and heavy breathing. I am my body. It is my carrier, my pleasure zone, my work of art. I must give it a holiday by treating it like the magnificent creature that it is. It supports me, gliding forward into the day with long strides. It houses my brain, my pumping heart, and my muscles that lift a pen or a telephone. *My body is my temple*, the old Bible adage. I must give it a permanent holiday, unrelenting protection. I must be its advocate and promoter. I am it. I am at the center of my own life. And I must find the psychological tracks, the mental restructuring—also a part of my body—to create protection and promotion of this self I find me inhabiting. Clear. Logical. My body lives in perpetual holiday.

These were my findings.

And these were my solutions. Since the moment at the Christmas table involved fear, desire, throwing it all to the wind, and, generally, a "giving up" thought, I had to think before I reached the table. I had to have a plan—a plan that recognized the panic of needing to overeat and being unable to stop. I had to create a scene that involved psychological and physiological actions.

This food-day plan must leave me satisfied in the area of food and people. First, food. I knew the amount of food I should have during that day. Any balanced weight-control program lays out weights and measurements clearly, so I decided to pack up my own combinations of salads and vegetables (often what I referred to as "fodder") and carry those with me. I would learn from my family, in-laws, or friends—wherever the party was taking me—what proteins or meats would be at the center of the feast. I would ask about how the meat was cooked, whether it was broiled, baked, or in its own juices. I would ask, and when I was tempted to think *this is going too far; I shouldn't ask about what they're serving*, then I would counter the thought with *this is my body, and it is that seemingly small item of how the meat is cooked that creates the very situation that is now urging me to ask. I must ask. Who else is going to take care of me?*

With plastic containers filled with massive salads or vegetables cooked in the microwave or boiled in water, I went forth. Often, if I was in the mood and knew that the main meat would not satisfy, I created three or four large sandwiches out of my day's prescribed amount of protein and light bread. On Thanksgiving, I'd bring the bread and then add their turkey. During my weight loss period, I would easily eat ten slices of this light bread in a day and still lose weight. The point here is that I organized my food to be present during the middle of the mind-battle, the center of the food frenzy, the celebration. I was proud of the massive bags that I carried into my parents' home or my in-laws' home. I would also work out in firm numbers what splurging casserole I might imbibe. I would ask the casserole cook what ingredients she had used, and then I figured, calculated, and wrote it down in a food diary that I considered one of the most essential tools of my program. I came to understand that "writing it down" was a beauty treatment. Literally. Keeping a record was one fundamental act, and this, in conjunction with several other tools, filled up my makeup bag for beauty.

Nineteen years have passed since those casserole Thanksgivings and chocolate chip Christmases when I recognized and worked out the elements that allowed me to manage my body. Since then, here in Dubai, another aspect of balance has surprised me. It even shocked me at the beginning. This is my ability to take a day— probably once a month—to eat what I want and when I want. When I first took this day and kept no record, and purchased on a whim, all the foods I lusted after, and ate at will—including potato chips, candy, croissants, mango juice, mayonnaise, butter—what I wanted just at that moment—I felt fear. Back to the old out-of-control and start-over feelings. But this didn't happen. I filled quickly and just stopped. The next morning, I felt satiated both in mind and body. I didn't have to feed my "mistake" because it wasn't a mistake. I took out my half-sheet of paper, wrote down my meals for the day, hung it on the refrigerator, and felt full. Full beyond the urge that wants splurge. What surprised me was my ability to return to my fine machine of order that filled me with its shift of food, to my time of the day that allowed me to think of other things during the day without running away and covering stress, pain, and unpleasant feelings with food. It's as if I had my cake and ate it too. This knowledge of emotion and a recognition of the series of days trailing behind me in which I'd lost weight and maintained weight; this acknowledgment that I had done this, that I could feel the range of human emotion, too; this habit of feeling it all and allowing emotion was the key. An open day is healthy and human. It does not equate to error.

Full—to feel full. Fullness is more than food fullness. The fullness of food lasts a short time and must be fed again. It gets full, and then there's nowhere else to go. That was my problem at the beginning. Fullness came soon, and there was nothing else to do but lie there and let the body do its work, digesting, pushing it all through, so I could fill it up again. But fullness could instead be fullness of the whole scheme—that is, my life. The same mantra. That mantra is wise, and it is habit, bare old unphilosophical habit, that provides fullness. And habit occurs through my mind—turning thoughts back to what I am, to what I want. Words first. They build *me* and make *me full*.

A second element of this fullness occurred when I fixed food—that is, when I hung around my miniscule kitchen, concocting recipes that included all my new knowledge of proteins, fats, and carbohydrates. I figured and cooked. I broiled and cut. I enjoyed the division of my dish into four or six portions. I enjoyed wrapping up each square of my finished product and covering it with Saran Wrap and foil. On the top of each little bundle, I'd mark in calligraphy the number of proteins, fats, breads, and fruits contained in that luscious handmade treasure. I enjoyed tucking it into my tiny freezer. These bundles were jewels. They would give me my five o'clock filling and a life of thin thighs. I made them tasty. Potatoes with mushroom soup, broccoli with cheese, tastes from my childhood: allspice, nutmeg, cloves, and cinnamon. I chose foods that evoked my past and prepared them with attention to detail, measuring light margarine and broiling away the fat in hamburger before I turned it into my burrito.

This engagement with food was part of the fullness. It was a delicate operation, tasteful and elegant. I danced around my kitchen like a queen, generating my jewels, shining them up.

Malls, Mercedes, and Makeup Bag

There's no other way around it: the malls of Dubai are works of art. The standard comment, intellectual and foreboding, that crass urban sprawl will be the doom of the globe, doesn't work here. These edifices are monuments to human ingenuity. What could be more reasonable than a glittering gathering place in the desert that contains a five-star restaurant, Missoni, Armani, Harvey Nichols, Tiffany, and a ski slope? Add fountains and gardens engineered into an interior oasis. Etch it all in marble and mirrors. Add Cinestar's fourteen theatres, Virgin, and Borders. Build the exterior with domes in pastel green and lavender. Provide grand multiple entries from parking lots—and you have the fabulous work called The Mall of the Emirates. Malls are masterpieces in Dubai.

The Ibn Battuta Mall chronicles the medieval wanderings of one Tunisian explorer, Ibn Battuta. Countries the man passed through between the years 1325 and 1360 dictate the colossal interior sections of this mall. The China Court houses a full dowel with sails and barrels, deep red pillars, Pizza Express, and I-Max. Tunisia offers wandering streets with a painted smoky blue night sky. India presents a twelfth-century mechanical clock and a full-sized elephant with *fakir* who lowers and raises his arm to drop weights into a trough, marking the hour. The magnificent blue-and-gold tiled dome of the Persian Court rises over Starbucks, and Gloria Jean's beans tempt pedestrians ambling between the painted Osiris columns of Egypt's bright red and yellow corridor.

The Madinat Jumeirah is a North African *souk* without dirt. You wander through alleyways and small corners covered in dark wood beams, seductive Arabic music drifting between the eaves. All of this opens onto a waterway fronted by first-class restaurants offering global cuisine. *Abras* pull up with passengers from a linked hotel, the Mina A'Salam, and the Burg Al Arab looms its metallic sail over the canopies of Toscana, an Italian restaurant edging the terrace on the water.

The Mercato Mall is Venice with Ponte Vecchio and the Grand Canal and, daily, I'm alerted by the scene out my window of the even bigger and, yes, biggest mall in the world, growing mushroomlike around the base of the Burg Dubai, the tallest building in the world.

Disney World can't touch this place. Dubai has outdone Walt. Let the world scoff at opulence and conspicuous consumption. The phrase "too much" comes to mind. But I can't help thinking of Pericles declaring that Athens was the "school of Hellas" because Athenians balanced beauty with practicality. "We have not forgotten to provide for our weary spirits many relaxations from toil," he offered twenty-five hundred years ago. "And the style of our life is refined."[8] If you mix Pericles with Khufu, who built big, the Great Pyramid, and didn't hesitate to put it out there—then why not Dubai? Tourists troop to the Acropolis, ten deep at the Parthenon's linked fence; no one can keep the crowds back from the hucksters circling Cairo's stones on camels and horses. Dubai is the current copy of large vision, and humanity seems to need it. The world wants somebody to build big, go over the top, and show what we can do. We want an icon for our human spirit. It is where, a thousand years from now, grandpas with kids on their shoulders, mothers with strollers, and enthusiastic historians with guidebooks will crane their necks to see a column of mirrors and a shard of glass in the desert.

Dubai was here.

I've always wanted a Mercedes. Before I came to Dubai, this tank of a car represented to me steady, mechanical prosperity. A large well-tuned machine that could be polished and would stand through the years, a sturdy sculpture, practical and elegant. I bought one—an old blonde one with a wonderful pedigree. Not knowing anything about cars except their pleasing shapes and aesthetic acceptability, I was surprised when I looked through the Sunday pages of the *Columbus Dispatch* and discovered in tiny print boxes that many people were unloading these icons of wealth for small prices. I called. I accepted a date with a seller and wandered, planning to be a wise, bartering type, to the condo, where the woman's voice had directed.

The woman, a nurse, efficient and kind, revealed her reasons for releasing the car to me. Manual shifting had become difficult for her because of a recent onslaught of arthritis, and her husband had his own wheels. When their garage door eased up, I was stunned. There she stood, the blonde beauty of my wildest imagination—boxy, shiny, a standing silver emblem perched on her hood. She even had a feather duster in the back to swish off her leather seats. And to top it off, she'd been owned by a Hollywood producer. Her journey to Ohio seemed mythical.

I learned to maneuver four on the floor and barged around town for a year before I accidentally allowed the oil to run out. One morning, she stood unmoving beside the five-minute sign at the post office. I got out, still holding my mail, stared for a while, and then walked around the corner to the gas station.

Mike Hostetler and I trucked back and, within minutes, his head peered around my tank's magnificent hood. "Froze up." He covered her innards with a slam of his gloved hand.

"Froze up? What's that mean, Mike?"

"The engine's froze up. It'll have to be replaced."

My Mercedes fantasy lay scattered like broken glass at the foot of the five-minute sign, and the image of my clever, bartering self dissipated like Ohio fog over the post office as I watched Mike hoist the blonde beauty, crippled, onto his truck.

She stands now, silent, in my garage, her feather duster gathering dust in the back window.

I didn't keep her tuned up.

Now, in Dubai, with its labyrinthine twelve-lane highways packed with Mercedes (latest version, no vintage here), Jaguars, BMWs, Bentleys—I don't know their mechanical glories, only their association with days of languid wealth, relaxation, and speed—I remember my car, sitting, still, in the garage. I remember my Gatsby-like feeling of elegance and beauty. The unreachable reached. And I think how much more central to my life and elegance is the maintenance of my body. Cars and bodies. I could drive around all day long in a Bentley and not be beautiful behind the wheel, but instead be an overeating dowager, smiling, pretending in my cream puff explosion, as I spread across the leather seats.

Body first. This is the maintenance, the tune-up, the shine that I want and that I put first. All other accoutrement are just that—extra. When morning comes in the window and carries my eye over the desert, when I take the elevator down to my sturdy Pajero, when I slide behind the wheel, switch on the air-conditioning and back out between yellow convertible VWs and mint green Jaguars, I know I'm going to the right place—to the beach to tune up my body. The walk, the stretch, the morning talk to my inside mind. Tuning up the inside and shining up the outside.

Maybe someday I'll get my Mercedes fixed, but she's a

secondary machine. The wizardry of this flesh, its interlocking bones and muscles, are my passion.

Counters with rows of regenerating creams, exotic pyramids of pencils for brow, lid, and lips, tall chairs with elegantly, smooth-skinned women leaning over faces sculpted in pinks and tans, and caches of crystal bottles glinting in blocks of gorgeous, hope-filling, eye-holding beauty. I love it. To enter a department store cosmetic display is celebration. Estee Lauder and Ralph Lauren are Paris, Rome, the world, adventure and art, alive in beauty's industry. I collected all of the black-and-white Lancôme makeup gift bags in the eighties, and why not? We are here to want to be beautiful. We are here to make our bodies into exhibitions of our lives. Sackcloth and ashes for some, but not me, although I do believe the adage "beauty begins on the inside." However, my insides tell me I'm allowed to want this exterior beauty, too, and if I want it, there are behaviors I must learn first. These behaviors I consider the tools in my makeup bag.

First, I record. If it is food that tempts and plumps me, it is food where I begin. Taking the elements of current nutritional knowledge, I know I must take in so much protein and fiber to live. I have looked at various charts and plans and know I must have protein, fat, vegetables and fruits, and carbohydrates. At the beginning of each day, I write down on a half-sheet of paper what I should eat to maintain my weight. I know that five ounces of protein, three servings of fat, five servings of fruits and vegetables, and four slices of bread will keep me where I want to be. When I was losing weight, I ate exactly the same groups of food but reduced the servings of proteins and bread.

As I was losing my weight, however, it occurred to me that losing, maintaining, and gaining weight are incredibly close operations. Even with two Bounty Bars, a hunk of cheesecake, and a half column of sour-cream onion Pringles (they, too, are protein, fat, and carbohydrates), I was still eating almost the same amount as when I stayed the same on the scale or watched the metal marker move to the left. Joyous day—it was close. And if that was true, then I could make small adjustments to get to where I wanted to be. So the grim specter of years in self-denial, a lettuce leaf lying silent and lonely on a white plate, did not have to be. I simply needed to eat less in certain categories, and these categories and adjustments needed to be determined when I was rational, clear, and sailing along. For me, that time is in the morning. I laid out my plan in the morning so that when the doldrums and fatigue of afternoon and evening set in, I would simply follow my plan. When people have suggested that they couldn't possibly take the time to figure this out and write it down, I have told them that it takes less time to keep records on a half-sheet of paper than to spend hours searching out stylish plus sizes at Wal-Mart. I opt for the half-sheet and hangers with "small" and "medium" marked at the top. First beauty treatment: I strategize during my optimum mood hours.

Second, I have my food in place, ready to go. I value my food supply more than clothes—and I love clothes. During the last nineteen years, I have kept the right food accessible in my home, from the readily available cans of beans, carrots, asparagus, to the low-fat and low-calorie meals bulging in my small freezer. I keep a supply of low-cal yogurt. I have fresh bread. I love bread, and I make sure that I'm not eating stale crusts. I have my tubs of low-fat margarine, and I buy the best grapes, bananas, mangoes, papayas, strawberries, cherries, and oranges I can find at the grocery—in Ohio or Dubai. I do not scrimp here. Lovely fruits and breads satisfy me and, thus, they must be available when the balance of the day swings low. Shopping for these elegant elements of my makeup bag is a pleasure. I know when I see the latest pyramid of peaches or pears at Kroger that these luscious shapes *are* my beauty. They delight my mouth, and they make me slender.

Third, I move my food-time to the part of the day when I need it. This small adjustment is one of the greatest tools in the bag. I have talked, marveled at, and been generally fascinated by human beings' up-and-down times during a day. I've met afternoon people, late-night people, and my own kind—morning people. Who can say why we peak and descend when we do, during twenty-four hours? But we do. Early on, I realized eating was a frantic comfort, and I needed this comfort as the day waned, the mood kicking in about 2:30 or 3:00 in the afternoon. So by 5:00, I was usually a wild woman, not caring what I ate. I reasoned that if all of this occurred day after day, no matter what seemed to be the norm for most people, then I would have to revamp, according to my pattern. I needed food, mounds of it, in late afternoon; I simply had to move my feast to this crazed time. That's what I did. And do. I save my cache of delights for 5:00. Bread, often six slices, spread with margarine. One or two pasta meals. A mango. A bowl of cherries. An orange. Half of a banana. A dish of eggplant, onion, and peppers cooked in tomatoes. Whatever I write down on my half-sheet in the morning is what I spread out in front of me at 5:00.

I've been asked "no food the rest of the day?" When I was losing weight, for breakfast, I ate a vegetable—perhaps broccoli, cauliflower, or asparagus. I ate no bread and no fruit other than tomato. My favorites were saved like jewels for an afternoon food orgy. The vegetable was a filler with excellent nourishing qualities. Who said we have to have toast and eggs in the morning? Or bowls of cereal? Or pancakes and waffles and bacon? I ate my vegetable with joy; actually, I came to feel little interest for food in the morning. In past years, when I was at various stages of losing and planning and trying, I ate a slice of bread, a teaspoon of margarine, and one lonely egg. But I always wanted more and, by 10:00 in the morning, I had determined that I would have more. And more. And more. This usually evolved into doughnuts, as many as I could wolf down, before the disgusting binge breathing set in.

Since the dark mood kicked in around 2:30 or 3:00 and I actually ate at 5:00, I was left with several hours of potentially dangerous low energy. But my mind knew that if I could last out two or three hours of afternoon ennui (my cave time), on the other side would be a feast, and I would be full. In the early days, if I had eaten the prescribed one slice of bread in the morning with the half-grapefruit, I would have felt deprived, not getting all I could have, the max, the spread of stuff later—and then mid-afternoon became a kind of waiting for more deprivation. But knowing at 2:30 that everything I really desired awaited me, that earlier I had eaten only brilliant green broccoli and lush cauliflower or asparagus—well, the realization was overwhelmingly simple and profound: I could have my cake and eat it too. In other words, I filled myself, and I lost weight by shifting according to my emotional variations. Week by week, moving my food to the time when I needed it caused me to lose weight. One-half pound, one-fourth of a pound, two pounds, week after week—I was filled and lost weight. That replacement of food by time was an essential, simple, and sophisticated tool in my makeup bag. Nineteen years later, here I sit, at my computer, slim, knowing that this evening I will eat until I'm full.

I worked out a plan based on my needs. I looked at the pattern of my eating and adjusted my schedule. I was pragmatic. In the past year, I have altered my morning and noon schedules to include some protein and carbohydrates. This adjustment now works for me, and I'm able to continue my modified behavior. Walnuts, oatmeal with honey and raisins, and low-fat milk sustain me during the morning without setting me off to binge on doughnuts. I accept this small portion of food as part of my health regimen. I see myself on the path, moving.

Each person must realistically survey her day—the excuses, the tension, the non-thinking grab—whatever she knows she is doing—and then adjust. You should do that with everything in your life that you want to change. You alone can make the decision to find what you need. When haranguers suggest that I shouldn't be eating my big meal as the last meal of the day, I answer, "This is what I need. See my slender thighs? They got this way because I know what I need." When others have said they couldn't possibly get through the first part of a day with only vegetables, I suggest they try it or alter their proteins to fit their needs. Each person knows her irrational moments; she can judge. She is the one to take care of herself.

The fourth tool in my makeup case is movement, a small program that I've kept in place for these past nineteen years. Maybe you're saying now, "Oh, here we go. I knew there'd be exercise. Yeah, yeah, I know I have to do it, but look at the things I've started. And stopped." Let me say upfront that I'm not an athlete, in the sense of engaging in strenuous, organized sports. But my reasoning tells me I must move. Move or die. Move or get crotchety. Move or increasingly detach from life, increase pain, and just plain allow myself to not manage this most precious encasement—my body. When I set out my plan for word change, I incorporated this language into my body movement; I talked while I walked, or rode, or touched my toes. I talked out loud: "I am moving toward my goal weight, and I am beautiful." Verb tense was the key. I spoke in the present tense, proclaiming that, at that moment, I was moving. At that moment, I was beautiful. At that moment, I was strong. Nothing should wait for another day. It had to be now, and "now" is possibly the most important word in my word hoard. Love now; lose now. Life does not pause.

We are here and whole. No matter what emptiness of spirit or fullness of overeating we feel, we are whole. And wholeness exists in the present. The multitude of self-help books out there on the market, in addition to the wisdom of ancient texts, declare that the present is where life is.

At least twenty years ago, I read Shad Helmstetter's *What to Say When You Talk to Yourself*, and it was in those pages that I learned the "present tense" trick.[7] That small shift in word form, from the future "I will" to the present "I am," created and continues to shape the quality of my life. Simple logic. I'm not trying to be perfect, pushing toward that quickly dissolving mirage in the distance. I am perfect. On my outdated stationary bicycle, looking out on my green Ohio hills, or on my old Schwinn, zooming down the road between cornfields, or on my feet, walking along the jetty out into the turquoise Arabian Gulf, I repeat: "I am moving to my goal. I am beautiful, strong." All is present tense, where it should be. Words sing through our brains like chants, spells, or magic. And that's what they are. Words change things. Magic.

So I move, and I talk. And just like the placement of food at the time I need it, I place movement at the time I know I will do it. Morning. Even when my mind is filled with stacks of papers I must mark, clothes on the chair I must hang up, and piles of bills I must sort, I move first. My program involves a series of stretches and strengthening exercises and the bicycle or a walk. Each person can put together her own program, but whatever it is, she must work for her own success—locate this essential tool at a time that she continues to keep in place, when she knows she will do it. The habit sets in, and she will come to enjoy this indispensable tool in her makeup bag.

Beach

June 11, 2004

I experience the exotic daily. On weekends, from my stretch of sand, the Gulf slides out to the horizon in slate blue. Roosters crow, and calls to morning prayer shimmy in the air. I press footprints in the beach, moving down to the edge where the current play of water changes with the magnet of the moon. This morning, my space between water and walkable sand is narrow. And, because it is before dawn on a Friday, shadows form pockets of people at intervals along the white-edged blue. Charcoal smoke and a soft, glimmering red spot gather in one group of shadows, and my closest route to the waves takes me past a figure that resolves itself into a man sitting in a plastic chair next to a dull fire. He is as close to the water as he can sit without being carried out by the next thud of mane-shaped foam. He doesn't turn to look at me as I pass within a foot of his hand. Because the tide is in, the beach is small and tilted, and shells crackle under my shoes.

First, I walk toward my line of rocks, boulders stretching from yacht masts into the sea, where a light blinks green, off and on, as a warning. I see the same stretch of horizon, but with different configurations, each morning. At a fallen fence, I turn, anxious for the day's frame on what I know will rise fantastically out of the mirrored water, jutting into an Arabian morning. A massive sail, clad in mirrors and steel, its side fluid in silhouette. The Burg Al Arab, Tower Arab, the only seven-star hotel in the world. Easter Island heads, the Great Pyramid at Giza, the Sphinx, cloud-topped stones at Machu Picchu, rocking gondolas in Venetian canals—and now the Burg, the latest installment in the human imagination, something out of a science fiction *Thousand and One Nights*. It is mine, in this moment on the beach. I am there, walking toward one spot on this day in the year 2004, glutting myself on a beach fire and the monolithic celebration of the human mind rising out of the water before my eyes.

Closer, my feet still struggling with the sand, I pass three women in *abayyas*, sitting on a blanket, and three bobbing bodies just offshore. The women laugh, talk, and look out at the men. One calls in a language I cannot understand or speak. Farther up, I pass a runner, an Indian building his thighs, disciplining his life under the same spreading scene, a building shaped like a sail, and its companion wave, the Jumeirah Beach Hotel. A wave and sail, huge, mine, human and spectacular, with my own flesh moving between nations, safe in the world. In Arabia.

June 18, 2004

On this morning, I set out to record what gives me peace. Dubai. By 4:30 AM, I have driven from my tower out to the weekend beach. Even though the sun hasn't made its raging appearance over the day, the water appears light, the world on the Gulf dimly lit. I park, take one last swig of water, and open the back of my Pajero to stuff the plastic bottle in with other recycling. I turn to the sand, pass a young man on the wall, dip my shoes in the soft pull, and scuff down to the water. I bathe in the gray early morning and soft sounds from other beach people. On my way down to the fence and yachts beyond, I pass no one walking, but a man and woman are sitting on a blanket to my right and farther on, I hear regular snoring. Three men are stretched out under the night. The beach is a living room, a bedroom, a kitchen. People live here successfully because there is no fear. No robbery. No threat of death. I reach my rocks and turn, and there before me looms the metal sail in the sea. I pass a man in white robe and prayer cap, the same man I saw yesterday, with the same walk, same determination, heading toward the fence, turning, just like I have done. A muscled Indian man runs around me. Faces take on distinct features in the rising light. Four women, pulling up black robes above their ankles, laugh in lacy waves. A father, a mother, and three children lounge on a blanket. One of the kids, a plump boy, jogs off, down the beach.

The day is my feast. I know my excellent fortune: I walk here in Arabian sand with the whole world around me. I teach, but, most of all, I learn. When I have made my second turn, moving back up toward the wall and my car, I try to think of words that could paint the luxury I own. I could have gold and pearls from this City of Gold, where men fifty years ago dived off dowels with no air equipment to harvest oysters' beads. I could have ten tailors stitch up any design, Italian, French, in several days. I could eat in a new restaurant each night, with elegant, gracious service and food like works of art and still not go through the dining list for months. But the greatest luxury speaks in quietness. I can walk on this sand with all the people of the world. We can laugh and talk and pass one another in the dark. And we are not afraid.

Horses

Horses. Big and sleek. Arabia has horses, of course, but the phrase "Arabian horses" didn't register fully for me until I arrived in Dubai. Although my dad had built a beautiful barn on our Ohio land that became his Arabian horse farm, I was not a horsewoman. In my twenties, I tried to ride and did—fitfully—but not naturally. So the horse, a mythical creature, remained an idea for which I required no spurs, no pungent leather saddle, and no trembling flesh.

When I first saw horses in Dubai—full-sized, metal—lunging out of the tops of villas on Jumeirah Beach Road, I was stunned. Later, I saw gold horses grouped at the entrance to the Royal Mirage Hotel. And one evening, I forced myself to Nad Al Sheeba, the horse track, and watched evening crowds gather around the rush of dust as this delicate power roared by. But the incident that punctuated the inseparable connection between Arabia and horses for me occurred one morning during my walk.

In half-dark, just past the lighted high tent coverings on the beach and under a full moon, I saw movement beyond the white surf. Lights braided in and out of the palms along the walk, but I still could not make out the motion in the waves, a plate of sea with filigreed edges roaring onto the sand. Walking nearer, faster, to see perhaps a desert Loch Ness, I was stunned, caught high in my chest with recognition. Horses, riders in the sea, plunging farther out. Brown gloss against black-blue painted sea with a slice of moon.

"How beautiful. How beautiful," I said out loud to the palms and rocks. "How beautiful."

Down into the sand, I pushed toward several figures standing, only shadows on the shore, they, too, looking out at the horses in the sea. A man, turning to me in the dim light, said, "Good morning."

I held my hand out. "Hello, I'm Sandy."

"I'm John. Out for a morning jaunt?" British, I registered. We both kept our eyes on the water where those otherworldly animals galloped against the waves.

"Beautiful. What is this, John? It's so magnificent and … and strange. These horses in the sea before daylight. With riders."

"The sheikh's stables. They love water. Just like children." One rider pulled back the reins, her horse whinnying wildly, raising its front legs above the sea. "She's edgy this morning. She's not been feeling well."

I realized that "she" was the horse and that this world I was witnessing took in the attitudes and the comfort of all those perfect sculptures. Children, sleek, magnificent Pegasus, looked after and draped in luxury. I watched, hypnotized by the odd juxtaposition of clothed riders on animals swimming in the sea. I watched until three horses met the sand and walked like beautiful, unconcerned models to a van with a blue light flashing. Self-absorbed and elegant children, pampered, living richly simply by being alive, these animals. Their beauty inbred and fading only with injury and age.

John, a former jockey, became a friend during the cooler months when his keep wandered for morning play down to the Gulf. A trainer, John's blood rolled with the blood of horses. I could see on other mornings how the riders, young men and women, barefoot, without saddles, and John, were a league, inseparable, needing one another, taking to the Arabian Gulf on winter mornings in Dubai.

Here

Think of the consummate folly of attempting to go away from here*!
When the constant endeavor should be to get nearer and nearer here.*[9]
——Henry David Thoreau

When I pad barefoot around my apartment in the morning, glancing out my window at lights outlining the length of the Emirates Towers, running water on my dishes from last night's supper, pulling up the cover on my bed, hanging up a brown jacket left on the chair, I know no second is a throwaway speck. Common acts are holy. They're activities setting up the day before me, motions sweeping up the day behind me. They will never come again. I think of a prisoner choosing his last meal or a hospital patient facing news that only a few months or days are left, and I rehearse what shifts of mind will occur when the door to the other side appears ahead. Most crucial for my life is the ability to remain, fully decked out, in the moment. Now. Here.

The sweep of time can be tolerated if we mortals eye something in the distance, preparing it now and here—a meal with the right china or napkins, the band concert where our child is playing her flute, a door opening on that first date with a new man, a new house, a new dress, a new recipe. The moment skids and whirls, lifting us up in thought toward the future. And if we attend obsessively and meditatively to peeling the sweet potato or waving to our child from the front row of the gym, then we can live. But when we wake up to see a space between our cuticles and the red nail polish from last week's manicure or mold on a lost vegetable pushed to the back of the refrigerator in its plastic container, we flinch. They have passed. That broccoli and paint were last week's accoutrement. We loved them. We looked at them. We planned with them.

For whatever we do to still the moment with paint, we rise up in the wind of time. Like Dorothy whirled away home, we will go there. We might as well go in style, our bodies portable art, our attention on that other who rides the day with us. "You're wonderful, my darling girl," I tell my daughter when I can, as she studies for her degree. To fit into a form—of words. Essays—the profile, the travel piece, the position paper—arbitrary forms for a moment in time.

"What's that, Miss?" I've just made my last swirl with a yellow star and stick figure whirling on red feet. Star and dancer appear with the Arabian Peninsula, a piece of the world, sketched on a white board in Room B036, on the desert, Dubai.

"That's you, aaah—what's your name?"

"Fatma, Miss."

"That's you, Fatma, and us. All of us now—in Room B036, Ground Floor. Nowhere else. Here, the most important moment of your life. Not the second you walked in. That's gone. Not the minute you walk out. It's not here yet. Just now. The most perfect. We're dancing."

"And over there, Miss?" Fatma points to a matching star over a flurry of lines far to the left, the west of my map.

"That's West Liberty, Ohio. My home. And that's my daughter dancing with us. Now. The same moment. Alive." I fling in the date—September 4, 2007—and color in DUBAI and WEST LIBERTY. I scroll up this fast map every class from that first day of the semester. I do it to let my students know and to remind myself that only here and only now count. And all that we do is arbitrary form.

We try to make sense of our hurtling lives by forms. "Only forms, my dears," I announce to my composition class on opening day. My students, their black robes glittering in the afternoon desert sun filtered through windows at the back of the room, sit upright, scarves pulled tightly around their heads. "They are collections of ideas, that's all. Rules laid out to make talking easier. To help us speak to one another on this hurtling rock ball we call Earth. And what's it all for anyway? It's for love." They nod, courteous and smiling. They understand the map and forms. They understand arbitrariness. They live in a shifting world where they select, with seriousness, ring tones for their latest version Nokias, where their teachers announce, "Here is a body of knowledge for the ancient Greeks—Pericles and Socrates. Learn it." They wait, restless, for their drivers and maids to pick them up under the desert sun; they hook up to Google to know what's showing at the Mercato cinema. They watch *Miss Congeniality 2* and *Troy*.

An essay introduction with its body paragraphs and conclusion, the formula I am bound to present to students, gives the illusion of control, but all rushes forward into evening and morning. The day and the essay disassemble and dissipate with the night. It seems to me that Plato had the right idea with forms, that grand chair, the perfect idea of *chair* out there in the universe somewhere, making all of our little chairs here on earth reasonable. Stephen Hawking, the brilliant wheelchair-bound British physicist, has suggested we're making it all up. Scientists and theorists across the globe debate the meaning of what appears to be waves, particles, and observed phenomena influenced and altered with our staring and our attention. Since Plato's cave, this question has haunted us: what is reality? I suggest that the only reality is the moment—all past and future dipping weirdly into the present—the perceived now. Form is our way to deal with it—the wild rush into aging. And form is not only a coping device with eternity; it is our skill, our talent, and our necessity. We create heroes for religions. We read about the latest divorce tangle of Britney Spears or Brad Pitt, our models to play with, criticize, and observe. We plan for the graduation party, the wedding, the PhD. We must do it to come to form, disentangle, and come to form again.

Sometimes, as I'm writing, I think I should form up something else, create a fictional simulacrum, a temporary land I weave from words, but I know the main character will always talk about now. The protagonist can do nothing but go back to her page with the knowledge of now. And she will dress up, arrange her dishes, and keep to the speed of words that must necessarily be stilled on white paper. All the heroines, then, will realize they are only forms and jump down from the page and take on flesh. The best ones will say, "It was for this. I go from here."

Mortality and joy lie next to one another but seem estranged. The lingering and mysterious nagging thought that you live, grow older, and eventually leave your body—the one you're working to enhance—appears diametrically opposed to the concept of joy. But because this duet is common and unalterable, a clear light shining on its frightening pattern, because it is outrageous, it is simultaneously wonderful, full of wonder. Consequently, I don't intend to take this flesh and chastise it for wanting beauty. The Spirit who created this grand plan has included the desire for form and balance, for patterns that engage a sense of symmetry or asymmetry, for bodies that drape textiles with grace, for skin that lies soft against sturdy muscles. This is not a mistake of sin-driven birth. This is the innate vehicle of women, men, amber ants building sand temples, and turquoise birds concocting twig pockets for eggs.

So I grab joy, the outrageous nature of life, and smile. And the second a stray thought wanders to "I didn't do it right," I dismiss those words, turn back to my path, and walk on up the way, talking out loud: "I am beautiful and strong. I'm myself now. Here, where I'm supposed to be."

Clothes

September 12, 2001, and Now

I can still see them—rows of black robes and black boxes, computer covers, rectangles, lining the tables before me. The room was cold, with the air-conditioning clanking frigidity into that space. Stark and utterly bare—our world that morning, September 12.

I think I brought my computer bag, empty, and laid it on the table. Was I mother, sister, teacher, friend, or fearful companion on this planet Earth? I was all, I told myself.

"My dears, this is a terrible thing. We must talk."

No one answered in the icy room. Only black on black with blank agony registered palpable misery between us. "I know you are stunned and afraid ..."

"Will you hate us, Miss? Will you hate us?" From the front right, the spot where Laila sat, came these cries.

"I love you. Never could I hate you." Their grief and fear

matched mine; to work, emote in a void of not knowing, was profound. But there was only one way through, and that was through. Keep going. We did.

Then, as one event followed terrifyingly on the next, a tsunami racking up another grief in another place, we kept going. In my tower, men at the desk packed up clothes for those sitting stunned on beaches far from the desert. Glass images cried across my TV screen. At the closet, the Emirates towers looming out my window, I shuffled through, seeing what I could send. I picked out clothes for myself. I laid them on the bed—my skirt, my sweater, my morning shoes. Clothes marked another day, some packed in bags and boxes marked "tsunamis" for others on torn beaches and some laid neatly across my bed for me.

When I returned to Dubai with my Bernina and its worn direction book, box of feet, bobbins, small screwdrivers, and my old red pincushion, pins and needles sticking in its sand-packed fabric skin, I returned with my friend. No matter what this barrage of equipment weighed, what lifting, grunting, awkward hurling of luggage it took after my bags rounded the belt at the airport, my sorrow was too great at the thought that I would leave my sewing machine behind. With this machine I had loved—overcast with its notched foot, flinging majestically, rhythmically, threads for Brooke's Dorothy costume on Halloween. Watching from my sewing room window, red birds sailing from spruce to pine, the foot sparkling, thumping in the sun of some morning, I had spun up webs that were more than cloth for my sister, my mother, and Dan.

And now, I recall my Great Grandma Sally's skirt, bonnet, and shawl, resting black and silent in my Ohio hall, proving that now for her was then, and clothes marked the spot. As fast as I write, the moments drift out over the desert, relentlessly, commonly. And I ask myself *what was it all for?*

Put it on, Sandy—those clothes. Mark your half-sheet of paper for the refrigerator. Go out. Down the elevator of your tower. Take this day. Dress it up—faux, facade, food, and flesh. Love.

It was for this. I go from here.

Epilogue:

Linear A

I unlocked Linear A
Last night
Today read with me
All language is black sticks on paper
Rock
Temple wall
All time a tick of clocks
Sand in glass
And means the same
This is the Museum of Me

The spotted flesh on this right arm
More Mystery than Schliemann's dirt
My foot in Ur
My knee in Crete
And Machu Picchu
Ha
Resume your mists
This statue walks
The clay still breathes
Its head displayed each time I go downtown

I click the channels off
Discovery
Remote control an artifact thrown on the bed
I open up a cupboard door
I take a cup
My brown-bean coffee spills onto the countertop
I touch this morning's bread
It's soft
Howard Carter, look
These things, these things.

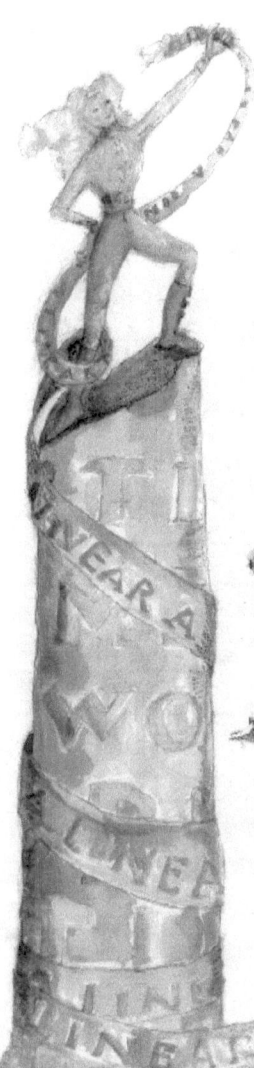

unlocked   Linear A
Last night
Today
Read with me
All language is black sticks on paper
Rock
Temple wall
All time a tick of clocks
Sand in glass
And means the same
This is the Museum of Me

he spotted flesh on this right arm
More Mystery than Schliemann's dirt
My foot in Ur
My knee in Crete
And Macchu Picchu
the
Resume your mists
This statue walks
The clay still breathes
Its head displayed each time I go downtown

I click the channels off
Discovery
Remote control an artifact thrown on the bed
I open up a cupboard door
I take a cup
My brown-bean coffee spills onto the countertop
I touch this morning's bread
It's soft
Howard Carter, look
These things, these things.

May 2003 — March 2004

Notes

1. William James, "Habit," *The Principles of Psychology* (Cambridge: Harvard University Press, 1981, originally published in 1890). <http://psychclassics.yorku.ca/James/Principles/prin4.htm>.

2. Freeman Dyson, "The World on a String," *New York Review of Books* (May 13, 2004), p. 19.

3. Henry David Thoreau, *Walden or, Life in the Woods* (New York: Harper and Row, 1965), p. 182.

4. Richard Carlson, *You Can Be Happy No Matter What: Five Principles for Keeping Life in Perspective* (London: Hodder and Stoughton, 1999), p. 44.

5. Daniel Goleman, *Destructive Emotions and How We Can Overcome Them: A Dialogue with the Dalai Lama* (London: Bloomsbury, 2003), p. 266.

6. Daniel Goleman, *Destructive Emotion and How We can Overcome Them: A Dialogue with the Dalai Lama* (London: Bloomsbury, 2003), p. 189.

7. Shad Helmstetter, *What to Say When You Talk to Yourself* (New York: Pocket Books, 1986), p. 76.

8. Thucydides, "Peloponnesian Wars," in vol. 2 of *The Humanistic Tradition*, ed. Gloria K. Fiero (Boston: McGraw Hill, 2006), p. 82.

9. Henry David Thoreau, "Nov. 1, 1858: Here," in *The Norton Book of Nature Writing*, ed. Robert Finch and John Elder (New York: Norton, 1990), p. 196.

Bibliography

Carlson, Richard. *You Can Be Happy No Matter What*. London: Hodder and Stoughton, 1999.

Dyson, Freeman. "The World on a String." *The New York Review of Books*, May 13, 2004, 16–19.

Goleman, Daniel. *Destructive Emotions and How We Can Overcome Them: A Dialogue with the Dalai Lama*. London: Bloomsbury, 2003.

Helmstetter, Shad. *What to Say When You Talk to Yourself*. New York: Pocket Books, 1986.

James, William. "Habit." *The Principles of Psychology*, 1890. http://psychclassics.yorku.ca/James/Principles/prin4.htm.

Thoreau, Henry David. *Walden or, Life in the Woods*. New York: Harper and Row, 1965.

———. "Nov. 1, 1858: Here," *The Norton Book of Nature Writing*. Edited by Robert Finch and John Elder. New York: Norton, 1990.

Thucydides. "Peloponnesian Wars," in vol. 2 of *The Humanistic Tradition*, edited by Gloria K. Fiero. Boston: McGraw Hill, 2006.